Hair

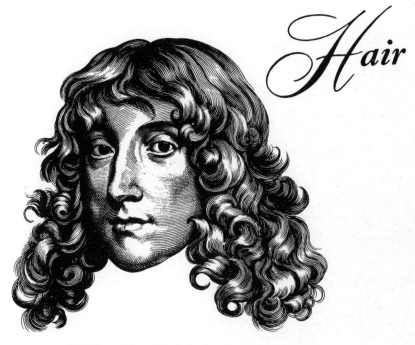

The Elector Palatine Charles Louis (1617-80)

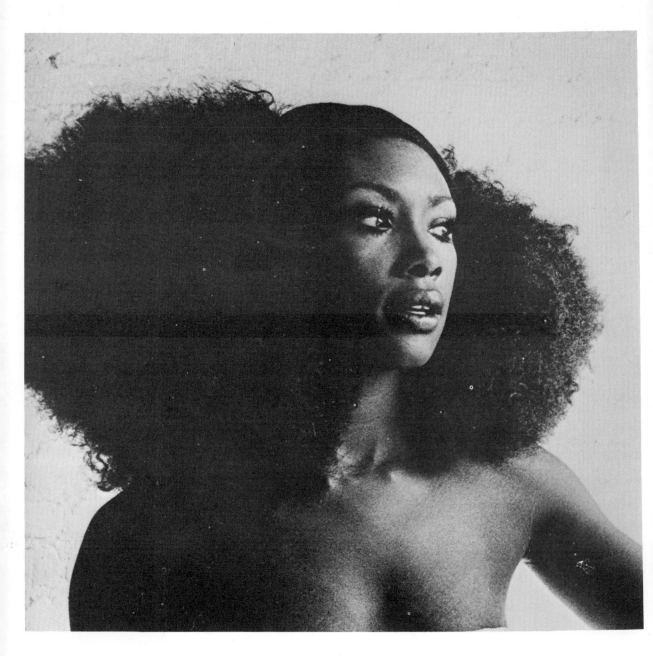

Even in hair styles, Afro-nationalism means "black is beautiful."

Hair

Sex Society Symbolism

Wendy Cooper

 Stein and Day/*Publishers*/New York

Editor   Roy Gasson
Design   Susan Tibbles
Assistant Editor   John Simons
Research   Michèle Rimbeaud

First published in the United States of America by
Stein and Day/*Publishers*, 1971
Copyright c 1971 by Aldus Books Limited, London
Library of Congress Card Catalog No. 70-167706
All rights reserved
Printed in Yugoslavia
Stein and Day/*Publishers*/7 East 48 Street, New York, N.Y. 10017
ISBN 0-8128-1429-0

Contents

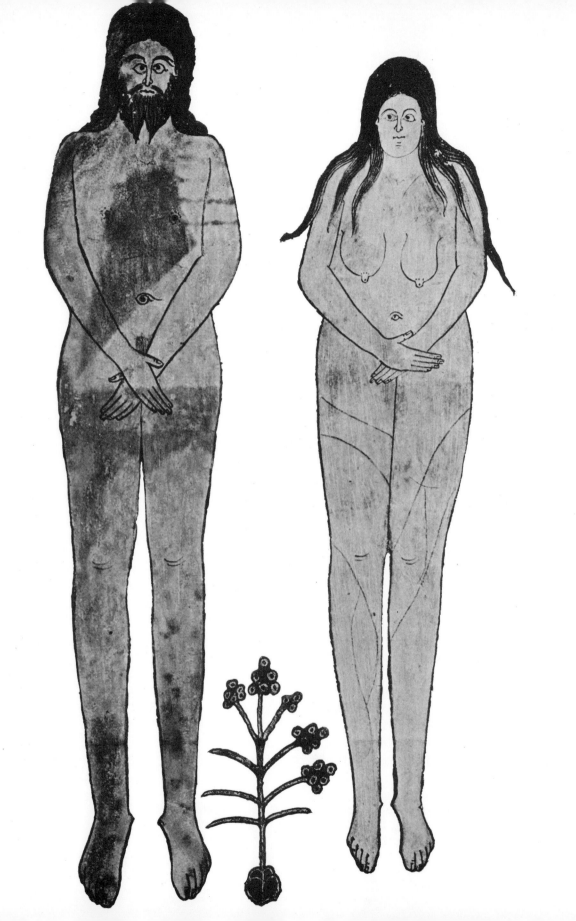

1 *The Nature of Hair*

As a species we exhibit an overwhelming preoccupation with our hair and—more sadly, in our later years—with the lack of it. From the earliest times of which there is any record, hair—its length, texture, color, growth, and loss—has exerted a strange fascination on the human race. It has woven its way into myth and magic, folklore and legend. Night-dark tresses and golden locks gloss the passionate outpourings of romantic poetry and prose. More prosaic forms of hair punctuate the sober annals of history, medicine, and the law.

Perhaps it is simply because man is the only "naked" ape that we have developed this obsession with hair. Had we evolved with as dense a covering of hair as have the other primates, we might have taken it as much for granted as we do our all-enveloping skin. Probably, it is the very distribution of our hair—the fact that it grows densely only on some regions of the body and, even more, that much of this growth coincides with puberty—that has invested it with a powerful sexual significance.

The fact that it can be cut and shaped, with a normally guaranteed regrowth to allow for changes of length and style, has added considerably to its charm for us and has made it not only a conveniently pliable form of sexual adornment and attraction but also an easily controlled variable to denote status, set fashion, or serve as a badge. It has become not only sexually, but also culturally and socially, significant.

All these aspects have become increasingly important as man has grown increasingly sophisticated, but it is the functional uses of hair that must have been vital to our earliest ancestors. A good covering of body hair could protect against extremes of heat and cold as well as against bumps, blows, and abrasions. It could offer a handhold to enable the young to

Adam and Eve, from an 11th-century French manuscript, show the characteristic male and female patterns of facial and head hair, but the artist has concealed their pubic hair, which also differs between male and female.

cling to the mother, padding against friction, and even a degree of camouflage. So the mystery is not why early man, like other primates, should have had so much hair, but why modern man has come to have so little. While other animals have retained their fur or feathers, why has the body hair of *Homo sapiens* become weaker, thinner, shorter, and finer?

Perhaps the simplest theory of hair loss is that some extrovert ape with a taste for adornment experimented with animal skins and so by accident discovered clothing and made hair redundant. Or it could have happened for a less frivolous reason. It seems probable that our ancestral apes were forced by an adverse climate and shrinking forests to come down from the trees to a less protected environment. More easily adjustable artificial coverings might then have been the answer to wider variations of temperature, so that gradually, over many centuries, the need for hair diminished and nature responded by allowing it to become much finer and shorter. Or did this weaker hair growth perhaps come first, for quite other reasons, so that early man was driven by increasing discomfort to replace his own natural hair with the pelts of dead animals?

And how about his discovery of fire? It has been suggested that this too may have contributed toward making a heavy natural fur coat superfluous. There could well be a connection, but which came first—fire or hairlessness? Man alone among the primates had the wit and will to discover fire and clothing, and man alone among the primates has lost hair to a marked degree. But the very discoveries could have been in response to urgent need, as so many of our technological advances still are today. Hair loss and cold may have resulted in fire and clothing, rather than the other way round.

We have to remember that evolution is not so much a planner as an opportunist. Probably many factors worked together, each additional advantage gained from hair loss confirming and strengthening the process. As a hunter, competing on the plains with fierce nocturnal carnivores better equipped in tooth and claw and speed, man would sensibly choose to try his lesser skill in the daytime, despite the heat. Armed with only simple short-range weapons, he would need both to undertake long-sustained chases and to make quick rushes to catch and kill fast-moving prey. By shedding his heavy hairy coat and increasing the number of sweat glands on his body surface, he was able to lose metabolic heat much more quickly. So—cooler, lighter, better able to maneuver—naked man had a better chance of survival.

The exposed skin brought other advantages. It was less liable to offer a breeding ground for parasites, and easier to keep clean and free of

Opposite: the princess in the tower lets down her hair for her lover to climb—a fairy-tale representation of a woman's ability to overcome impotence in the male. On page 10, a diagrammatic cross section showing hair structure within the skin (1, sebaceous gland; 2, arrector pili; 3, papilla; 4, hair bulb; 5, follicle; 6, nerve fiber). On page 11, the hair jungle—the hairs of part of a human scalp seen through a microscope.

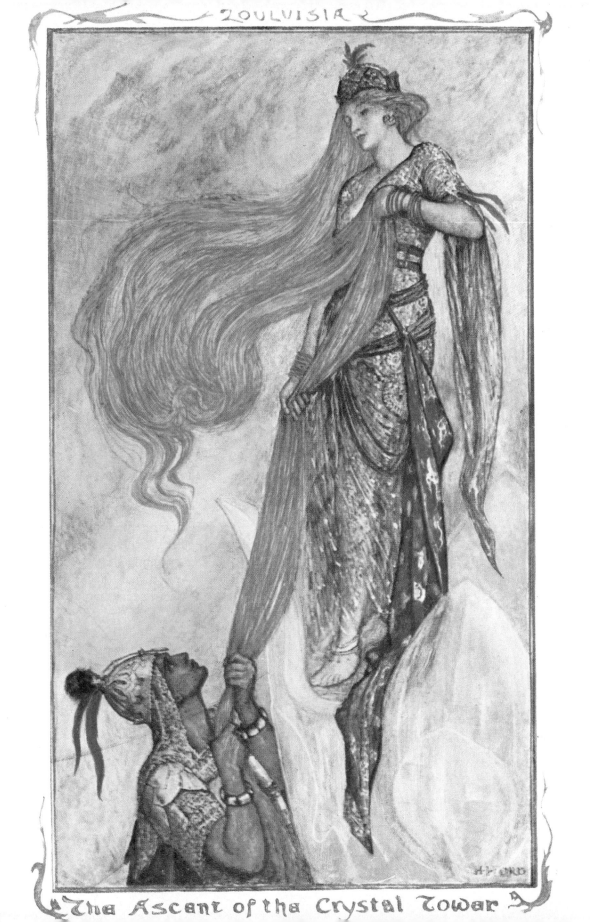

The Ascent of the Crystal Tower

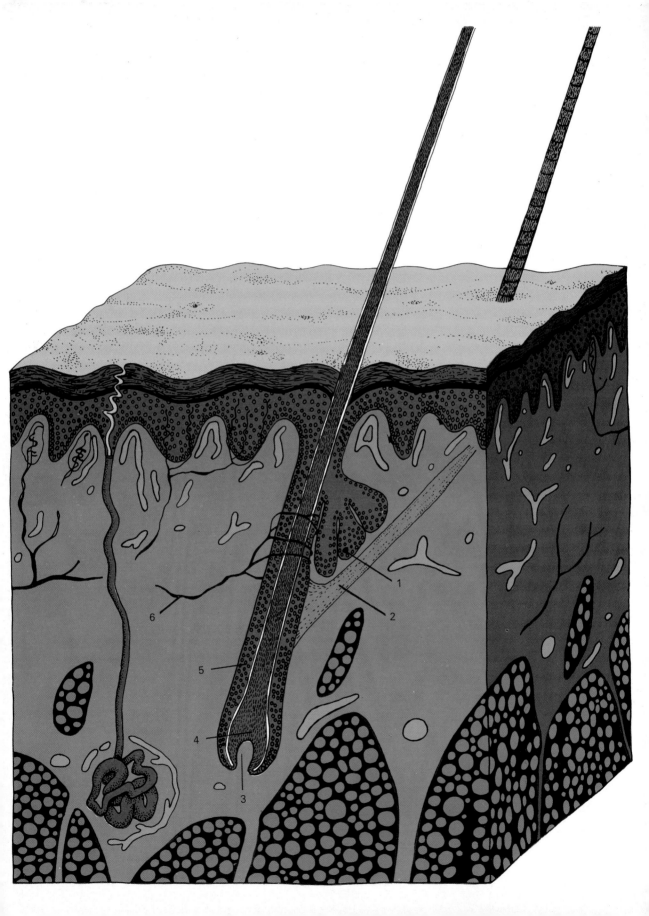

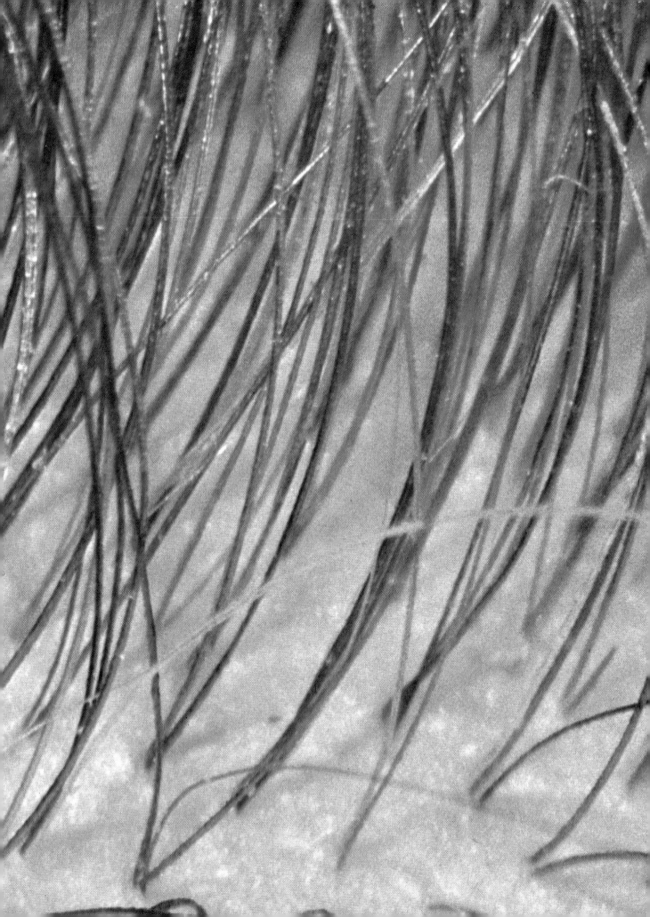

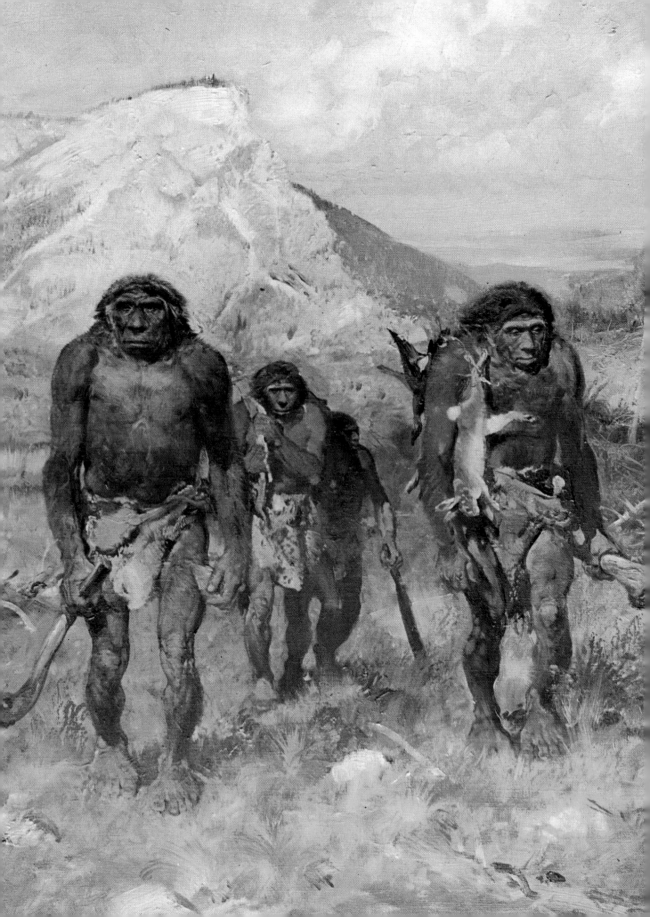

disease. It afforded a clear identification and signaling device, particularly on the sexual level. Male primates tend to be hairier than their females, and, by extending this difference, the more naked human female could well have gained in sexual attraction—a situation no doubt satisfactory to her but even more so to the species. Natural selection would then carry on the good work by tending to breed in greater and greater hair loss, affecting the male also to a lesser degree.

It may be presumed, too, that naked skin added considerably to tactile sensation, heightening sexual excitement and awareness between mating couples. In his book *The Naked Ape* (1967), zoologist Desmond Morris stresses the value of this to a species in which pair-bonding was important. Dr. Morris argues that the naked ape's survival depended on his success in transforming himself from a casual fruit-picking ape in the trees to an organized hunting ape on the plains. His success at hunting depended in turn on a high degree of cooperation between males, which had to extend not merely to killing the prey but to sharing it and carrying it back to the females and young, who, unable to keep up with the fast hunting pack, had to be left behind in home dens. Such a degree of co-operation could have been possible only if sexual rivalry was reduced to the minimum and the unprotected females could be left safe from the advances of other males. This, rather sadly, appears to be the utterly unromantic origin of the human need to fall in love, to develop a pair bond, and to remain faithful. And it relied for success not on any moral, ethical, or religious sanctions (though those were to come later), but on the power of sexual imprinting on a single person. Evolution may have favored naked skin for this reason.

Dr. Morris argues that man's prolonged childhood also strengthened the pair bond. The child, because of its long period of dependence, formed a deep personal relationship with its parents. The loss of this at maturity created a "relationship void" that had to be filled by a new attachment to a sexual partner. Perhaps for this reason or, more probably, to increase brain-power, an evolutionary process called neoteny developed in man, as in many other species. Neoteny means the prolongation of certain infantile characteristics into adult life. In our case it not only resulted in our longer childhood but also ensured that, although we become sexually mature around 12 or 13 years old, our brains go on growing and developing for a further 10 years. Many experts see the weakening of hair growth as a side effect of this neotenous process. Our nearest relative, the chimpanzee, has at birth a good head of hair but an almost naked body. If this condition were delayed by neoteny, as it is in man, the adult

Neanderthal Man, who lived in Europe some 70,000 to 40,000 years ago, had lost some of the hairiness of his earlier ancestors, but was still, compared with modern man, shaggy of head and body like his ape relations.

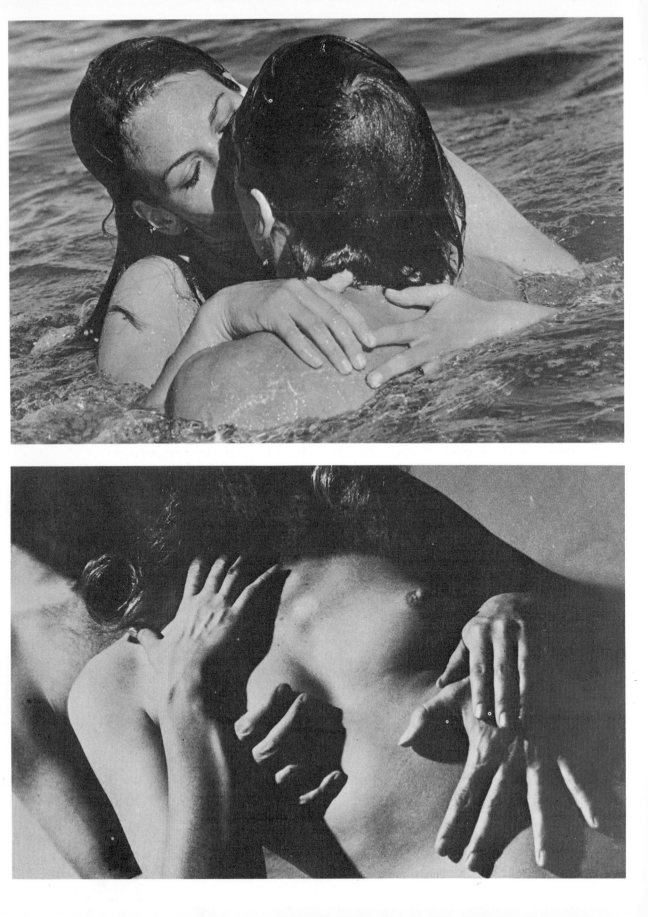

chimpanzee would have a hair distribution very like our own. But we can be sure that natural selection would allow a neotenous change only if it had special value to the species. So, although neoteny may explain how hair loss happened, we still have to puzzle among the various theories about why it happened.

One theory envisages an intermediate phase between fruit-picking and hunting, in which our ape ancestors moved to the seashore in the drive for food, and became aquatic. This explains ingeniously not only how we lost our hair (like the whale and other sea mammals), but also how we achieved both streamlined bodies and vertical posture. The theory sees us at first tentatively exploring rock pools and then, as we gained confidence, wading farther and farther out to sea until we had to haul ourselves upright on two feet just to keep our heads above water. Finally, we began to swim and dive for food. Then only our heads, still protruding above the water, needed to retain thick hair as protection against the glare of the sun. Eventually, armed with tools developed from those we used to crack open shells, we ventured back inland and began hunting larger game.

This intriguing theory, originally introduced almost frivolously as part of an after-dinner speech, has no real evidence to support it, but it neatly explains some odd facts. For instance, why is man able to make himself at home in the water and even enjoy it, while his closest living relative, the chimpanzee, dreads it? (Modern zoos utilize this fact to imprison chimpanzees on islands, cut off from freedom only by shallow moats.) Does the intermediate aquatic phase that the chimpanzee did not share with us account for this striking difference in our reactions to water? And what about the thick layer of subcutaneous fat we possess, for which there seems no satisfactory explanation? Unique among primates, did it develop—like the blubber of whales—to insulate us against cold seas? In particular, why does the fine hair on our backs lie differently from that of our fellow-apes? Directed diagonally and backward toward the spine, as if to follow the flow of water over a swimming body, is it a remnant of our early aquatic life, modified and streamlined to reduce resistance when moving through water?

But neither the aquatic theory, nor one currently being resurrected that we derive from bear-like ground creatures rather than tree apes, seriously upsets the most convincing reason for hair loss to emerge from the welter of speculation—that once man became a daylight hunter on hot tropical plains, he had to develop a means of losing metabolic heat rapidly. The wide distribution of sweat glands on the human body (modern man has between two and five million active ones) gives strong support

Top: love in the water. Perhaps because he went through an aquatic phase during his evolution, man—unlike the chimpanzee—can enjoy the water and even find wet hair and wet skin an erotic stimulant. Bottom: Darwin believed that sexual selection favored a woman's body naked of hair, the texture of her bare skin being both more sensitive and more sensuous to a lover's caress.

to this idea. These glands, plus a surface of hair-free skin to permit maximum evaporation, add up to the most efficient cooling system possessed by any mammal. And it is significant that where little or no metabolic heat is generated, as in the scalp, evolution has permitted man to retain his protective hair covering.

In fact we are not nearly as naked as we think. Our only truly naked areas are the palms of the hands, the soles of the feet, the lips, the nipples, and some parts of the genitals. Though we may not welcome the comparison, as adults we have more hairs than the chimpanzee. It may not look like it, but that is because, except in a few special areas, our hairs are now so fine and short as to be largely invisible.

But it is these special areas of dense hair that provide the most fascinating mystery of all. We do not know with any real certainty why we came to lose hair; equally, we can only speculate on why we have retained these odd patches of coarse growth.

The head is fairly obvious. It needs protection, so there was everything to be gained by "keeping our hair on." Similarly, brows and lashes help to protect the vulnerable eyes, and the hairs across the open passages of nose and ears act as sieves against insects, dust, and irritants.

Pubic hair and axillary (armpit) hair are a different matter. Although they may also have a protective purpose as padding against friction, the fact that they both appear at puberty gives them clear sexual significance.

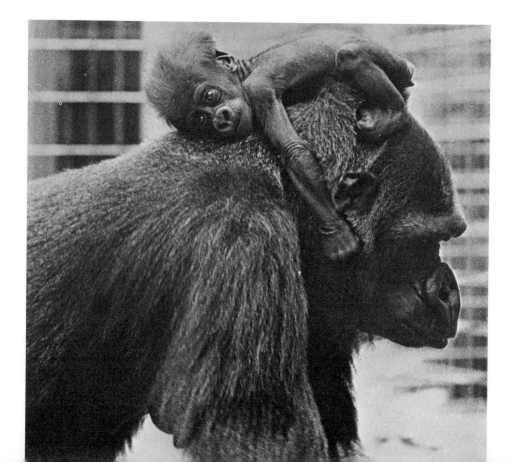

They are first and foremost signals of sexual maturity, but they almost certainly fulfill another sexual function. Both the pubic and the axillary hair grow in areas where the skin contains scent glands whose secretions need exposure to air to develop their full odor. The tufts of hair provide a holding surface for this oxidation, which releases a distinctive scent that serves—or, at least, served primeval man—as a recognition signal and a stimulant to sexual excitement.

But this explanation of why we have retained our pubic and axillary hair seems not entirely adequate. Nor does the theory that women kept their axillary hair for their babies to cling to during a stage in evolution when we were still partly tree dwellers and the mothers needed both hands to swing from branch to branch. The truth is that we do not really know. Our answers are based, at best, only on intelligent guesswork about the past, and on limited observation in the present. Both seem to confirm the role of pubic hair as an outward badge of maturity and a visual marker to the genitals. Pubic hair is a clear sexual cynosure.

So, with pubic hair of both sexes, we are probably on firm ground—sexual ground. We can stay there, with fair confidence, if we think of specifically *male* hair—that of the pubis, abdomen, chest, and back, and particularly the moustache and beard. Adult male monkeys have extra hair growth to form beards, moustaches, and manes, all of which they use to give themselves a fierce appearance in the threat displays and scuffles that establish sexual dominance. In other words this hair is—to use evolutionist jargon—epigamic hair, which means simply that it is related to sexual dominance. There seems little doubt that human male hair at one time had a similarly epigamic function and so had a selective advantage in evolution. The well-endowed male, displaying his strong hair growth to add to his ferocious appearance, was more likely to frighten off his more scantily equipped rivals and emerge the victor in the struggle for a mate. Even today, when expensive cars, well-filled billfolds, and well-cut suits have become in many cultures the contemporary symbols of sexual dominance, there are still some men who can display a growth of epigamic hair that would not disgrace a gorilla.

Charles Darwin, the founder of evolutionary theory, believed that natural selection favored not only epigamic hair in the male, but also contrasting nakedness in the female. He believed that our ancestors liked a woman with a fine head of hair but a naked body. (Because body fur had no functional use to make its retention necessary, this nakedness became assimilated to the male, who retained only his vital epigamic hair.) Certainly nowhere in the world do normal adult women have as much

A baby gorilla rides on her mother's head. Only a few days old, she has much the same hair distribution as a human adult. Human hair growth seems to be arrested, by neoteny, at what is merely a baby stage for other apes.

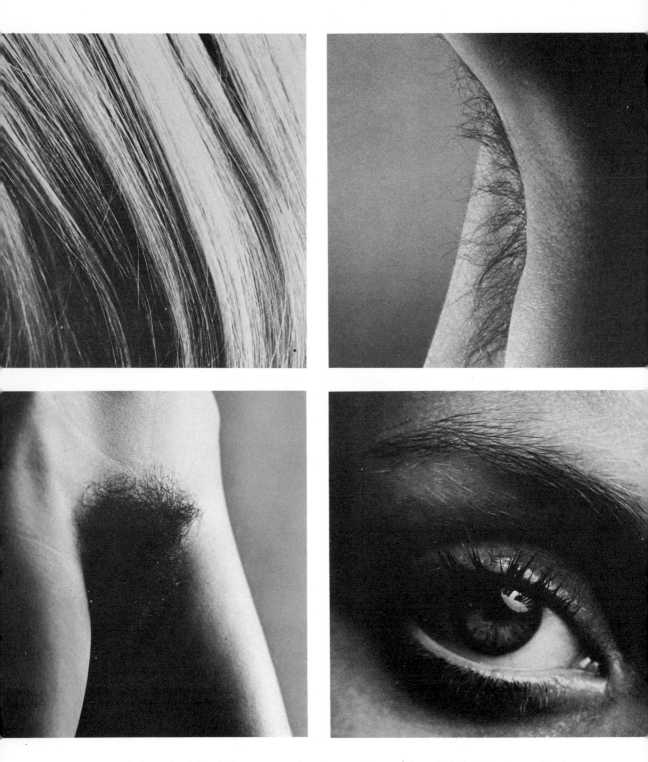

Evolution has left only four main patches of strong hair growth on the body of the human female— on the head (top left), in the armpits (top right), over the pubic area (bottom left), and around the eyes (bottom right). The function of these remaining patches of hair is still a matter for controversy—only head hair and the eyebrows and eyelashes seem to be purely protective.

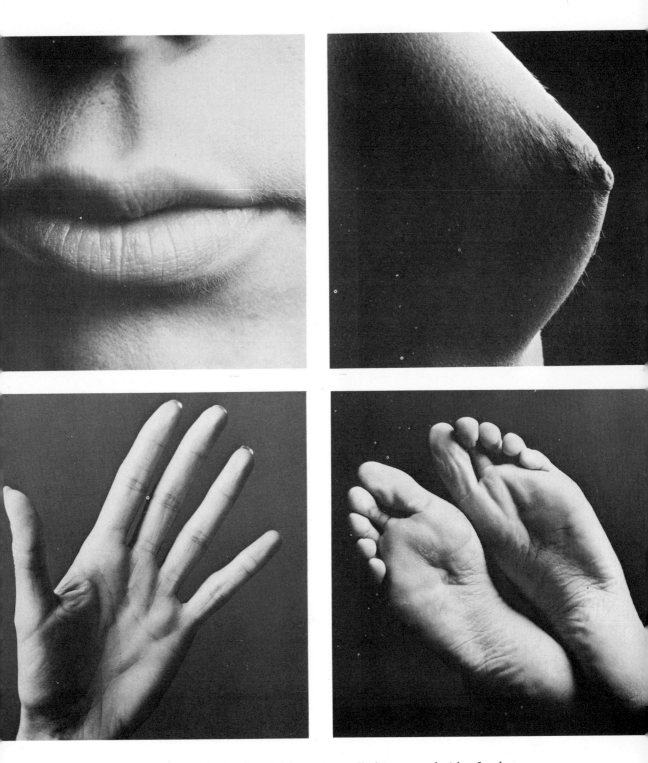

But the rest of the human body is far from hairless—almost all of it is covered with a fine down. Normally, the only external areas of a woman's body that are totally free of hair are the lips (top left), the nipples (top right), the palms of the hands (bottom left), and the soles of the feet (bottom right). These are all areas of extreme sensitivity to touch.

hair as men on face or chest, and this deficiency is known to be maintained by the hormone balance of the female body. It is only when this balance is upset pathologically or at the menopause that hair sometimes sprouts more coarsely on the chin and upper lip. And Darwin's theory gains support from our modern attitudes, for whereas most women do not object to hairy men—and indeed some find them especially attractive—many men quail at the very idea of a hairy woman.

So early man evolved into our familiar selves, with our few thick patches of hair standing out against the greater expanses of downy skin like thickets of long, coarse grass on a mown lawn. The hairy patches link us to the common heritage we share with our fellow apes; the barer skin differentiates us from them. Taken together, they add up to an odd distribution of hair that makes us immediately recognizable as members of the species *Homo sapiens*.

But we are not all alike, and racial differences—that too often in our history have given rise to suspicion, discrimination, and aggression—are apparent in hair. Hair, in fact, is second only to skin color as a physical sign of racial difference. Its texture, its color, and, to some extent, its distribution vary widely between different races. Almost all Mongolians (Chinese, Japanese, American Indians, and Eskimos) have straight *coarse* dark hair on their heads and only sparse facial and body hair. Negroes have slightly more body hair but crinkly or woolly hair on the head. The White races (Caucasoid) have an in-between form of wavy, curly, or straight *fine* hair, and more body hair than any other race except the Ainus—a primitive group (believed to be the remnants of a White people who once lived in Asia) that survives in the northern part of Japan.

The geographical distribution of hair color tends to follow that of skin color. People who have adapted to survival in strong sunlight, by acquiring heavier quantities of the pigment melanin in their skins as protection against excessive ultraviolet radiation, have both darker skins and blacker hair. Inhabitants of temperate lands have lighter skin tones and hair shading from brown to blond. Red hair, like the fair skin that goes with it, is dependent upon a deficiency of melanin (which in the skin is unevenly distributed into islands of freckles).

The pattern of hair growth, as well as its form and color, varies racially and clearly has adaptive value. Crinkly hair bunches into spirally wound locks, and really woolly hair clumps together in small spiral twists close to the scalp, leaving bare skin between the clumps. This may allow a greater area for sweating. The Bushmen of the Kalahari and the Pigmies of the African rain-forests both have tight spirals. The wiry mat-like hair

A Barnum and Bailey's circus poster of the late 19th century shows a troupe of Chinese acrobats performing while suspended by their hair. The act was possible because hair is strong—a single strand of Mongoloid hair has a breaking strain of about 160 grams. It is also elastic—it can be stretched by as much as 20 or 30 per cent before breaking.

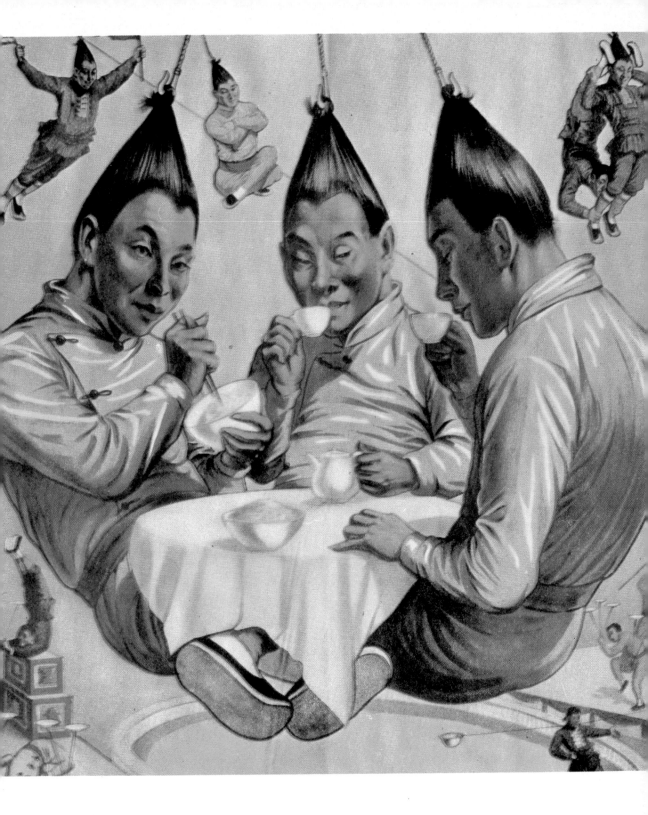

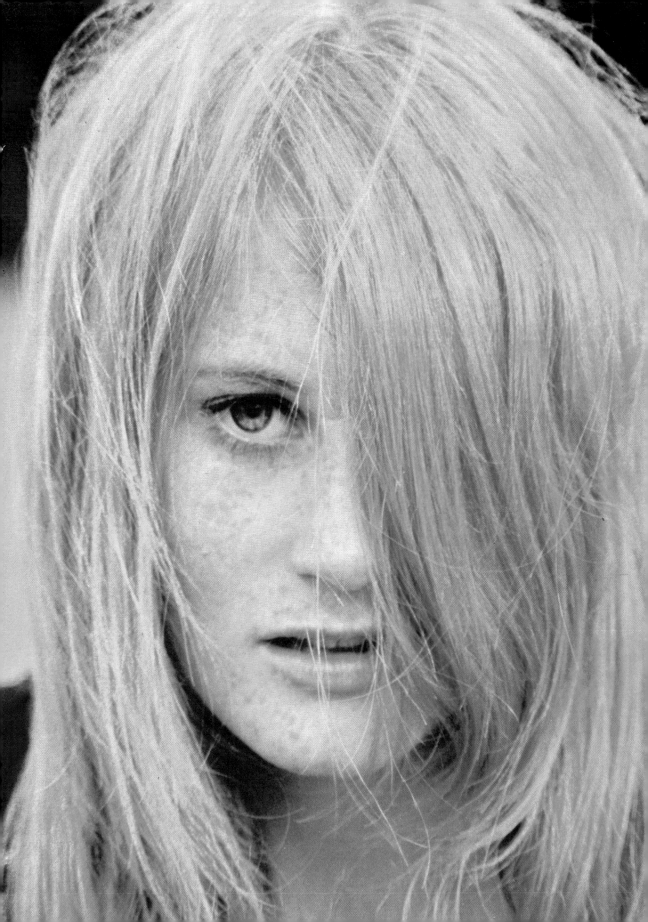

of some desert tribes appears designed to give maximum insulation. Of course there is nothing absolute about these broad divisions of hair type and color. Population migrations and interbreeding have introduced many modifications, dilutions, and mixtures.

Clearly anyone who has ever been tempted to think that a hair is a hair is a hair must think again. For hair varies widely not only in type, texture, color, and length between different races and between individuals of the same race, but even on the body of one person.

The unifying factor is that all these hairs, of whatever type, are produced from little pockets in the skin called follicles. These at least all start in the same way at the same time, if we go back far enough—back to the human embryo in the womb. Three months before birth, every hair follicle we shall ever have forms below the skin over the whole body— even the hair follicles for the beards and moustaches of adult men. This does not, of course, result in bearded babies. The facial hair follicles, like those for pubic and axillary hair, become fully active only at puberty, under the chemical impulse of body hormones. It is true that occasionally babies are born with a fuzz of fine hair not only on their heads but on their bodies also. But this is something quite different. It is lanugo hair, with which every normal human fetus is covered. Usually it is shed before birth, and replaced in the early months of life by fine "vellus" hairs, but occasionally babies are born who still retain it.

Each tiny elongated follicle, in which a healthy hair sits snugly, is far more than a mere container. It is a hair factory with the actual manufacturing plant, the papilla, situated at the base. This minute peg of tissue pushes up through the center of the follicle into the bottom of the hair, which grows around it to form the broader hair bulb. So the papilla is the nearest thing the hair has to a root, although the whole idea of a hair root is a popular misconception, for when a hair is plucked out, the papilla stays behind and simply starts manufacturing a replacement. Rich in minute blood vessels, it supplies amino acids that are synthesized into protein to feed the continuous formation of cells on the outer surface of the papilla. These new cells continuously being created from below push up the older ones, which, as they rise, undergo structural differentiation into the variously shaped cells that make up a hair shaft. After a final hardening process, called "keratinization," the shaft emerges from the mouth of the follicle as a visible hair. From its bulb-like base, the hair shaft tapers to a point at its top. It is the fact that these tapered ends have been cut off that causes a chin to feel stubbly after shaving. The notion that hair grows coarse and bristly after repeated use of a razor is a myth.

A natural redhead, owing the beauty of her hair and of her fair skin and freckles to a red hair-color gene coupled with a deficiency of melanin. The lack of melanin means that her hair is so lightly pigmented that the red coloring can dominate; it also means that her skin is only lightly colored except in the spots, or freckles, where the pigment has become concentrated.

Each hair follicle is supplied by one or more sebaceous glands, which produce oil to lubricate the hair, although their full function is not yet properly understood. It is the oil produced by these glands that gives the hair its gloss and richness. To each follicle is also attached a special muscle, the arrector pili. Downy vellus hairs lack this muscle (as do eyebrows), but often have large sebaceous glands. Hair muscles can be seen working very obviously and dramatically on cats and dogs, when fear or anger causes their fur to rise. In humans it is more normally a response to cold that causes the muscles to contract, producing goose pimples and up-standing hair. But in moments of great stress the same effect may be achieved through the body's hormone response. Our hair can stand on end with fear. Reports from World War II, for example, tell of memory-haunted men whose hair stood on end for several months after their experiences on the beaches of Dunkirk. A British army doctor, Sir Arthur Hurst, in his book *Medical Diseases of War* (1944), described similar cases from the trenches of World War I. "I saw several men suffering from the effects of severe emotional strain, whose hair permanently stood on end and could not be kept down by means of grease. In some cases I had the opportunity of comparing their appearance with what it was formerly, and the change from the sleek appearance when in civil life was most remark-able. One man, who kept his hair closely cropped, said his hair reminded him of the bristles of a hedgehog . . . . In some cases the hair of the body as well as the head has been persistently erect." The sense of terror shines through even the unemotional prose of the medical observer. Shakespeare made it explicit when the ghost of Hamlet's father said:

> I could a tale unfold whose lightest word
> Would harrow up thy soul; freeze thy young blood;
> Make thy two eyes, like stars, start from their spheres;
> Thy knotted and combined locks to part,
> And each particular hair to stand on end,
> Like quills upon the fretful porcupine . . . .

"Each particular hair" adds up to a great many hairs. A single healthy human scalp carries an average of 100,000 hairs, but there are wide variations from this figure. Blonds have as many as 140,000 hairs on their heads, brown-heads have about 108,000, and redheads fewer than the general average—only about 90,000. Each of these hairs (and every other hair on the body) is intimately connected with the whole physical being. Hair does not grow as an independent entity, like moss on a tree. It is an integral component of the body, as much part of us as our skin. Indeed, in some ways it may be considered an extension of skin; it is

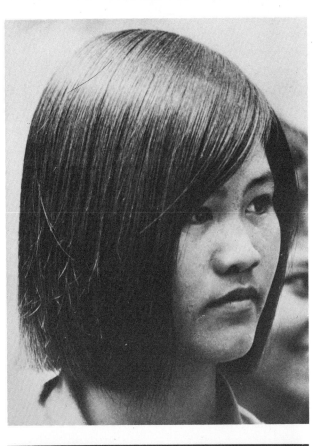

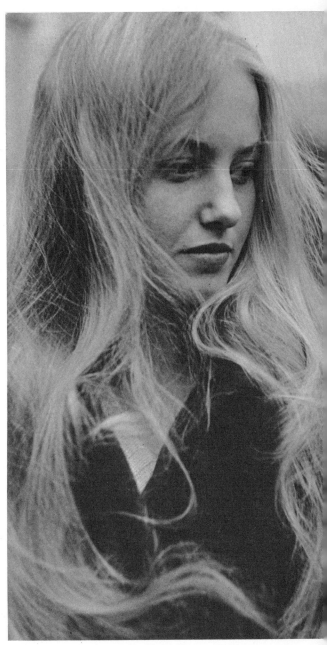

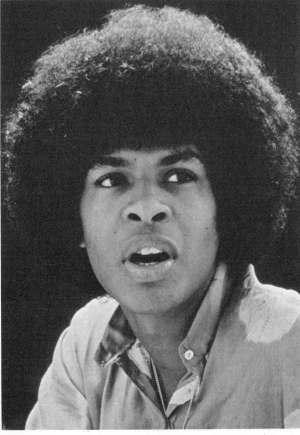

The three main racial types of hair. Above left, a Vietnamese girl with typical straight, rather coarse Mongoloid hair. Left, a young American Negro's hair has the characteristic woolly, tightly curled form classified as Negroid. Above, a Scandinavian girl whose hair is of the intermediate type known as Caucasoid, which may be straight, wavy, or curly, but is rarely as dead straight as Mongoloid or as crinkly as Negroid. The color of this girl's hair is also characteristic—blondness is almost always associated with Caucasoid hair.

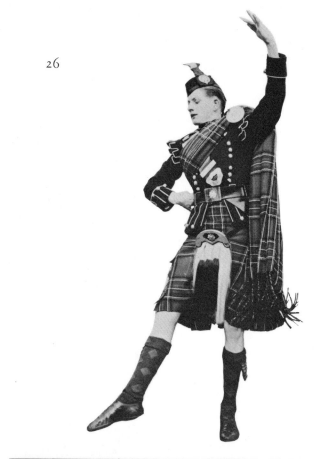

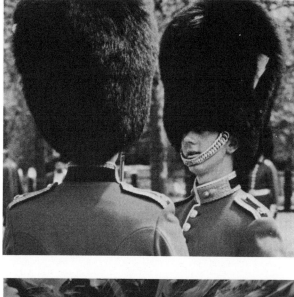

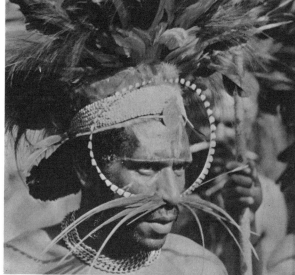

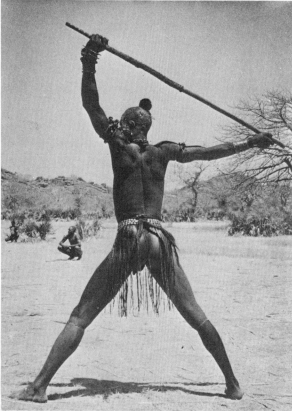

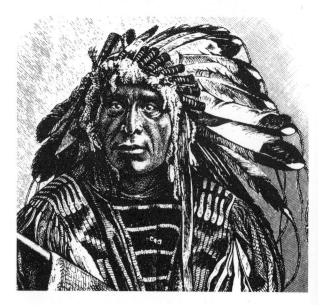

firmly linked to our blood supply and it reflects, as skin does, the general state of health of our body.

Nonetheless, hair growth is not a simple process, nor even a continuous one. Hair grows in phases. An active growing period (the anagen period) alternates with a resting period (telogen), and between the two is an intermediate stage (catagen), but the mechanism of this cyclic activity of the follicle is not yet fully understood. Certainly the duration of each phase of growth or rest varies, but we cannot explain why. Even to measure the *rate* of hair growth is not easy. It is very much an over-simplification merely to quote the usual figure of an average daily growth rate of 0.35 millimeters. Hair grows at different rates on different parts of the body and its rate of growth varies also with sex and age. Recent observations have shown that hair grows fastest when we are between 15 and 30 years old, and fastest of all in women between the ages of 16 and 24, who may make as much as 18 centimeters or 7 inches of growth a year. The rate of growth slows down still more when we reach our 50s. Hair growth also slows down during illness or pregnancy, although, particularly after a severe illness, it often compensates by growing especially fast during convalescence.

Contrary to a frequently held belief, neither shaving nor cutting accelerates hair growth—although, in some way not understood, both seem to prod lazy follicles into activity, so they may cause *denser* growth. But that hair grows faster in warm weather—a phenomenon often noted by regular shavers—is confirmed by scientific tests. Recently some evidence has been produced to show that the rate of growth of a man's beard is related to his sexual activity. His beard grows more quickly during periods when he has sexual intercourse than it does during periods of abstinence. Moreover, even the anticipation of intercourse is enough to make his beard grow. This discovery was made by a scientist whose work forced him to live in isolation and celibacy on a remote island during the week and to return to the mainland and normal life at the weekend. Over a period of several months of this routine he weighed the shavings from his daily shave and graphed the results. "The cycle is unmistakable," he reported in an article in the scientific journal *Nature* in May 1970. "The Friday peak comprises an anticipatory response during the day and the effect of intercourse; the increased beard growth falls off by Sunday, and by Monday it becomes smaller than on any other day of the week." He found also that, although sexual relationships seemed to have the most obvious effect on beard growth—"even the presence of particular female company in the absence of intercourse, after a period of abstinence,

Early man's abundant hair was an animal sign of sexual dominance—it had an epigamic function. Modern man recaptures ancestral memories of epigamic hair through substitutes—such as the sporran worn by the Scots guardsman (top left) and the skirt, made from human hair, worn by the Sudanese tribesman (bottom left). Similarly, the bearskin helmet of the British Brigade of Guards (top right), the ornate headdress of the Chimbu-man of New Guinea (center right), and the plumage of the Dakota Indian chief (bottom right) are all substitutes for a virile mane of hair.

usually caused an obvious increase in beard growth"—other factors were involved. Tension, anxiety, nervousness, excessive mental fatigue, and alcohol consumption were all associated with increased beard growth, whereas physical exercise and—contrary to other experimenters' findings— "high ambient temperatures" seemed to inhibit growth.

Even if neither shaved, nor cut, nor plucked, a hair still has only a limited life before it falls out naturally and is replaced by a new shaft. In animals the hair follicles all work together in synchronized activity, producing a seasonal, overall molting. But human follicles work more or less independently of one another, so that hairs are continually being shed and replaced, a few at a time. (This is just as well for our social habits and conceits, not to mention our ideas of beauty—although "I'm sorry, I'm molting" would make a splendid excuse for refusing the unwanted invitation.) Normally we lose anything between 50 and 100 hairs from our head every day and the life span of any particular hair is unlikely to be more than six years and may be as little as two.

The average length to which a hair grows in its lifetime if left uncut is 22-28 inches (55-70 centimeters). But averages are almost meaningless in this context because of the possible permutations of varying rates of growth with varying lengths of life. It does seem in general true that the lifetime of a woman's hair is about a quarter as long again as a man's. For this reason women tend to produce longer hair than men, but even in women it is rare to find hair more than about 3 feet (90 centimeters) long. Rare, but by no means unknown. In America the seven Sunderland sisters toured with the great Barnum and Bailey show in the 1880s under the billing The Longest Hair in the World. The sisters—who were rather plain country girls—had thick brown hair that hung down their backs and brushed the floor behind them as they walked. The combined length of hair that they displayed to the audiences of their singing and dancing act was said to be 36 feet 10 inches. Even so, the Sunderland sisters had to yield second place to a certain Miss Jane Owens, who at about the same time was exhibiting hair 8 feet 3 inches long. But the record for the longest hair of all time has been claimed, surprisingly, for a man. He was an Indian monk, Swami Pandarasannadhi, who was reported in 1949 by the *Toronto Morning Star* as having hair 26 feet long. This is about the length of hair each of us would have on our heads by the time we were 50 if our hair grew continually and never fell out.

Of all the popular beliefs about hair and its growth, the most macabre is the myth that hair goes on growing after death—a myth that is reflected in several "hair-raising" stories of coffins being opened to reveal lush growths of hair on long-buried corpses. Perhaps the most detailed of these stories is that told by a Dr. Wulferus in a letter written in April 1680 and published in the *Philosophical Collections* of the British Royal Society in the following year. Dr. Wulferus had been told that the body of a woman buried in Nuremburg 43 years before had recently been disinterred and he sought out the sexton who had been present at the opening of the grave. The sexton told him what he had seen. "The corpse lay the lowest of three in the same grave, there being two other corpses over it, the ground, bones, and ashes of which being removed, this coffin began to appear; through the clefts of which much hair was thrust out, and had grown very plentifully, in so much that 'tis believed that the whole coffin may for some time have been all covered with hair. The cover of this coffin being removed, the whole corpse appeared perfectly resembling a human shape, exhibiting the eyes, nose, mouth, ears and all the other parts; but from the very crown of the head to the sole of the foot covered over with a very thick set hair, long and much curled. Which strange sight (they never having seen the like before) much amazed the sexton and his companions; but he after a little viewing of it going to handle the upper part of the head with his fingers, found immediately all the shape of the body to fall, and left nothing in his hand but a handful of hair, there being neither skull nor any other bone left, unless it were a very small part of that which they suspected to be the great toe of the right foot. This hair was somewhat rough at first, but afterwards it grew very much harder, and of brown red colour . . . ." Dr. Wulferus sent a sample of the hair to the Royal Society.

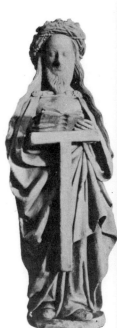

A similar "strange sight" was described by a doctor from Iowa in the *Medical Record* for 1877. In 1862, he wrote, he had attended the exhumation of a man who had been buried two years before. "The coffin had sprung open at the joints, and the hair protruded through the openings. On opening the coffin, the hair of the head was found to measure eighteen inches, the whiskers eight inches, and the hair on the breast five to six inches. The man had been shaved before being buried."

The truth, if any, behind these stories is hard to establish. Because hair is an integral part of our system it would seem an indisputable fact that once death occurs hair stops growing. But we know now that death is a process, not an event. It is possible, then, that some slight growth of hair may continue for a short time after the heart has stopped. Add to this the fact that the skin contracts in death, so that the hair can *appear* to lengthen— a once clean-shaven chin showing signs of an incipient beard—and we have some basis for the belief that hair grows after death. Another ingredient to the belief may be premature burial. This can, and does, still happen

This statue of a bearded female saint stands in Westminster Abbey in London. She is Saint Wilgefort, a Portuguese princess who was betrothed against her will to a suitor she did not love. She prayed that she might become so unattractive that he would no longer wish to marry her. Her prayers were answered. She grew a coarse beard, which repelled her suitor. Wilgefort devoted the rest of her life to religion, and died a virgin.

today. It happened with unguessable frequency a few hundred years ago, when a cataleptic trance or similar state of suspended animation might be mistaken for death. When it happened, hair would continue to grow on the still-living body in the coffin, and if the corpse were later exhumed its finders might well see a greater growth of hair than they expected.

But it is a long step from this to the hair-covered body described by Dr. Wulferus. Was the doctor simply the too-gullible victim of a sexton prepared to tell a good story to anyone who would buy him a drink? Was the sexton himself deceived by a growth of fungus? Or can it be that the myth has a basis in fact, and that there are exceptional circumstances in which hair *can* grow on a corpse?

There have been stories also of hair not only growing but changing color after death. But here, too, the facts deny the myth. The color of our hair is dictated at our conception by the hair-color genes we inherit from our parents, which decree the amount and type of pigment our hair will contain. The thickness of the hair shaft (and perhaps its oil and air content) also affects coloring, but pigment establishes the basic color.

If the key hair-color gene decrees a heavy deposit of melanin in and among the hair cells, the result is black hair. A little less melanin produces dark-brown hair; still less, light-brown; very diluted, blond. Red hair is the product of a supplementary gene that produces a diffuse red pigment. If the red-hair gene is present with a very active gene for melanin, then the red gene will be completely obscured. Some people believe that a hidden red gene can show its presence by giving a special richness to black hair.

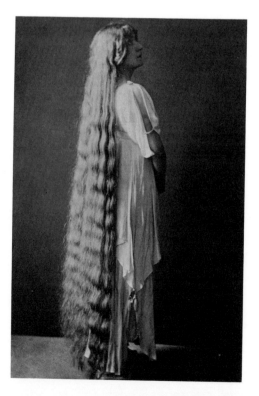

Right, a woman's hair allowed to grow to its full length —a photograph dating probably from the early 1900s. Such a mass of hair demanded a great deal of time and attention, which is doubtless one of the reasons why short "bobbed" hair became so quickly popular in the 1920s.

Hirsutism, or hypertrichosis, is the medical term for the condition in which hair grows strongly on parts of the body that have normally only downy, lanugo hair. Center, the "lion-man" Adrian Jefficzew from Russia, who was examined by the Society of Science in Berlin in 1873. Far right, Annie Jones-Elliot, one of the best-documented of bearded ladies. She was born in 1865 in Smith County, Virginia. At birth, she already had a well-defined moustache; her beard was fully developed by the time she was two.

Where the melanin gene is weaker, the red-hair gene shows up in reddish-brown or chestnut shades; and if the melanin gene is very weak, or absent, then true red hair will be produced.

Theoretically the red gene should dominate a blond gene that has laid only diluted deposits of melanin. But there are cases where blond parents produce a red-haired child, showing that one or both carried a submerged red gene. But with rare exceptions, the blond gene is definitely recessive to all darker hair shades. So the general conclusion is:

If you have dark hair you are carrying either two dark-hair genes, or one dark and one for another shade.

If you have blond hair, you carry two blond genes.

If you have red hair, you carry either one or two red genes, supplementing blond or brown genes.

Hair-color genes can be slow in asserting themselves, and light-haired babies often darken, although the darkening of hair with age can also be due to structural changes.

The graying of hair with age is a process of decolorization, with pigment, air content, and oil all involved, together with structural changes. Existing pigmented hair is not decolorized. Even removed from the head, hair keeps its color for hundreds of years, so it is not correct to think in terms of hair fading. But, as existing colored hair grows out, the new hair replacing it lacks pigment, and the mixture of this new white hair with the existing dark hair gives the gray effect. The time at which pigment-forming cells no longer transfer color to the growing hair is governed by heredity.

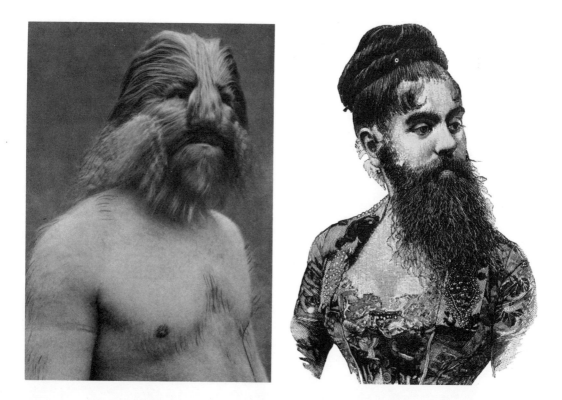

There is great controversy among hair experts about the cherished myth that hair can turn suddenly white with shock. Most authorities believe it to be improbable, if not impossible. Their doubts were not shared by the great Scottish writer Sir Walter Scott, who wrote:

Danger, long travail, want and woe
Soon change the form that best we know;
For deadly fear can time outgo,
And blanch at once the hair.

And, indeed, there have been reports of this phenomenon of sudden blanching. Most are pure legend, but there are medically attested cases also. A British army surgeon in India in 1859, during the aftermath of the Indian Mutiny, described the interrogation of a captured rebel sepoy: "Divested of his uniform, and stripped completely naked, he was surrounded by the soldiers, and then first apparently became alive to the danger of his position; he trembled violently, intense horror and despair were depicted on his countenance, and although he answered the questions put to him, he seemed almost stupefied with fear. While actually under observation, within the space of half an hour, his hair became gray on every portion of his head, it having been, when first seen by us, the glossy black of the Bengalee, aged about 54. The attention of the bystanders was first attracted by the sergeant, whose prisoner he was, exclaiming, 'he is turning gray,' and I, with several other prisoners, watched its progress. Gradually, but decidedly, the change went on, and a uniform grayish color was completed within the time named." Another report, detailed and well-documented, describes the case of a 38-year old Frenchwoman who in 1882 suffered great personal grief followed by severe financial loss. She became very ill, her menstrual flow ceased, and she had acute neuralgic pains in her head and shoulders. After two days of this, at 2 A.M. on January 30, 1882, her hair was still its normal black color. By 7 A.M. next morning much of it had turned white, and within two days she was almost totally white-haired. Her eyebrows and eyelashes remained as black as before. More recently, in 1947, the *British Medical Journal* reported a case of sudden blanching in a man aged 65 who, during World War II, had twice in one night escaped death by a hair's breadth in an air raid. By the next morning his hair had turned completely gray.

Dr. Agnes Savill, a British dermatologist and one of the greatest medical authorities on hair, admits the probable existence of this phenomenon of sudden blanching. She believes it possible that sudden and profound emotion may cause constriction of the vessels supplying the hair papillae, so that the cells are deprived of their nutrient and stop forming pigment.

But this could not affect existing hair, and a British zoologist, Dr. F. J. G. Ebling, has offered another explanation of apparent sudden blanching. He suggests that a scalp may bear a large number of white hairs while still appearing substantially dark in color. A rapid shedding of the dark hairs (which can and does occur) so reduces the proportion of dark to white hairs that the head appears to become whiter within a few hours.

Because laboratory experiments have shown Vitamin-B deficiency to be important as a cause of graying hair in rats, experiments with administering the Vitamin-B complex to restore color to human hair have been tried, with some claims to success. There is also evidence that the adrenal gland is especially concerned in melanin production and deposition, which suggests that stress is a factor in depigmentation. But, once again, we do not really know. For centuries medical science has tended to ignore hair, abandoning it to the quacks. So it is slightly ironic that, now that top scientists and doctors throughout the world are at last condescending to give it their attention, hair seems to be almost retaliating for past neglect by refusing to yield up its deepest mysteries too easily.

With the genetics of hair, though, we are on slightly firmer ground. Color is not the only inherited hair characteristic. There is the whorl, or manner in which hair grows wheel-like around the crown of the head. Some people have a clockwise whorl, others an anticlockwise one, and some 5 per cent have double whorls.

The character of the hair is also dictated by the genes. The woolly gene is the strongest; it dominates all the others. The crinkly gene dominates the curly, the curly dominates the wavy, and the wavy dominates the straight. An interesting sex difference has been reported, however, showing that male hair often tends to be wavier than female hair in the same family.

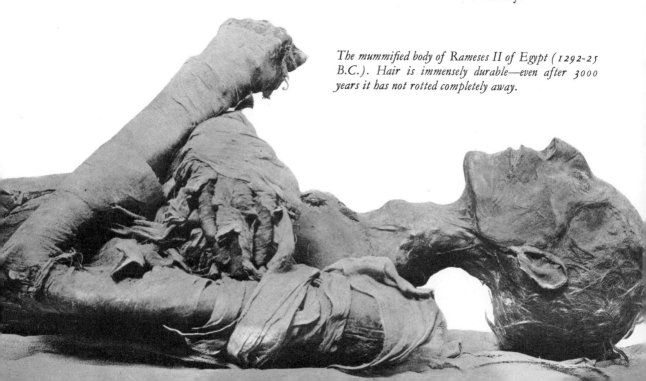

The mummified body of Rameses II of Egypt (1292-25 B.C.). Hair is immensely durable—even after 3000 years it has not rotted completely away.

It is an ironic state of affairs when one considers the agonies girls have gone through to acquire the curls or waves fashion dictated, and the equal agonies some small boys still suffer, scraping away with a wet comb to get rid of even the suggestion of a "girlish" curl. An exception to the dominance order is the Mongolian straight-hair gene, which may be dominant over that of woolly hair. But among Whites, the straight-hair gene is recessive to all the rest. It follows, therefore, that two straight-haired parents must resign themselves to having all straight-haired children. Parents with other types of hair will find prediction much harder.

With so many variables, it is not surprising that crime writers have sometimes allowed themselves to get carried away with the idea of human hairs providing their fictional detectives with firm means of identification. In real life it is not quite so sure or so easy. All the same, the Chicago police are reported to possess records of more than 150,000 different varieties of hair collected from criminals, and there have been real-life crimes when even a single strand has helped to convict a suspect. At Limoges in 1935, a mason, Pierre Bourget, was identified as the murderer of an old spinster by just one fair hair found at the scene of the crime.

Careful microscopic examination of hairs in a police laboratory will reveal characteristics of color, texture, thickness, appearance in cross section, and type of pigment, which all help in classification. Details of recent cutting, singeing, bleaching, dying, and perming—all of which produce recognizable alterations—can also be detected. Despite this, hair is not a totally precise means of identification. Too many people have very similar hair, and too often even hairs from the same head can vary.

But although hairs are not uniquely characteristic of one person as fingerprints are, or easily groupable as blood is, they are extremely useful for matching purposes; and they often play a big part in confirming or dismissing a suspect in a case, or in providing valuable corroborative evidence. However, their usefulness in crime detection is likely to increase dramatically with the perfecting of a new technique called "activation analysis." This makes use of the fact that the elements present in any material can be converted into radioactive isotopes by bombarding them with neutrons. The elements can then be identified by the radiation they emit. This method is so hypersensitive that it is possible to detect and measure radiation from incredibly minute quantities of material. So it is now possible, though rather expensive, to identify the trace elements in hair that result from individual food intake, personal washing and shampooing methods, local pollution, and environmental factors such as living and working conditions. This all gives a very much closer identification.

The hand of a modern man (left) compared with that of a chimpanzee. Although the man's hand appears to be much less hairy, it in fact bears almost as many hairs as the chimpanzee's. The difference is that human hairs are much finer and shorter and thus appear to be scantier.

Hair can also have a very special part to play in cases of suspected arsenic poisoning. Like the nails, hair absorbs arsenic. It can contain, weight for weight, more than any other part of the body; arsenic can be detected in hair when no trace of it can be found elsewhere in the body. The most famous case of suspected arsenic poisoning must be that of Napoleon Bonaparte, whose death on the island of St. Helena during his final exile, although officially ascribed to cancer, gave rise to rumors of foul play. Recently samples of his hair were submitted to activation analysis and it was found that the arsenic content was about 13 times the average.

A great range of sophisticated techniques can now be brought into play to make a single hair reveal so much. As well as extracting from it the secrets of all its inherent characteristics and any cosmetic treatment it has received, we can also tell—from the distinctive appearance of its end— if it has fallen out, or been cut, shaved, or forcibly pulled out in a struggle. It is perfectly simple to distinguish between animal hair and human hair, between body hair and head hair. And yet there is still one thing we cannot do. No one has yet found a way of sexing human hair. There is no way of telling whether a hair comes from a man's head or a woman's. It seems a curious situation, considering the strong sexual significance of hair and the important part the sex hormones play in its life and death.

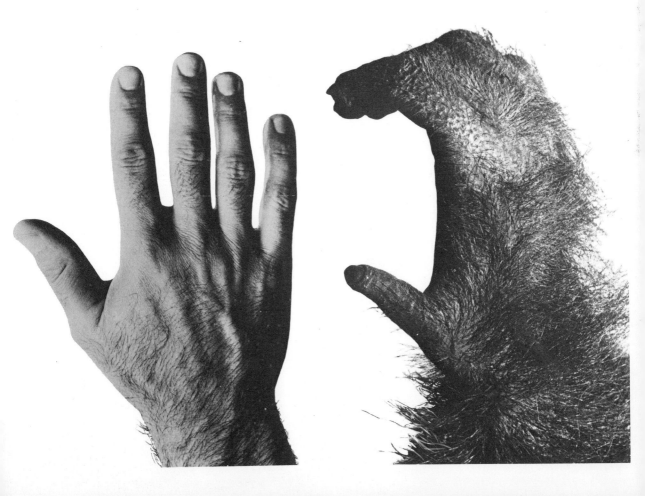

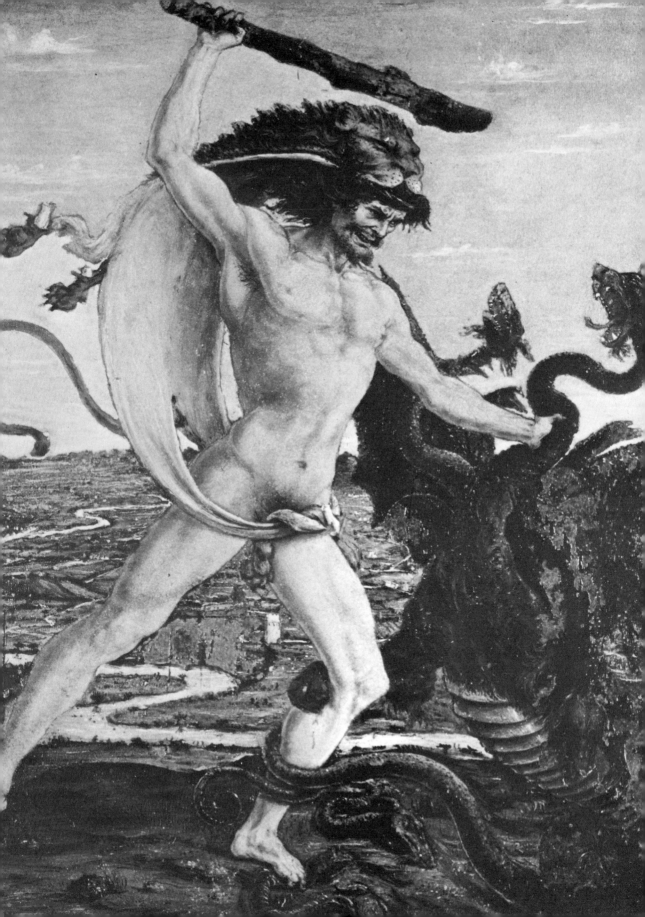

2 *Hair and the Male*

Men are hairier than women. They grow more facial hair. They have a stronger growth of hair on their chests and backs and, usually, on their legs and arms. Their pubic hair is longer, although finer, than women's and it is usually more extensive in area. A man's pubic hair grows up over his stomach, forming a triangle with its apex reaching toward the navel; a woman's ends in a more or less straight line above the mons veneris. So, because facial and body hair is one of the obvious characteristics that differentiate the male from the female, it is not surprising that hairiness has become a symbol and a proof of masculinity. The ability to grow a beard is a specifically male ability; a mat of hair on the chest is a specifically male possession.

Modern medicine, and in particular endocrinology, has now firmly established the hair-maleness connection by showing the vital part the sex hormones play in triggering the distinctive hair growth that accompanies puberty in the male. The growth of pubic hair usually starts between the ages of 12 and 14, when the development of testes and penis is already well under way. The downy vellus hair—already present but scarcely visible—increases in length, in diameter, and, later, in pigmentation. It gradually covers the pubic region and finally spreads toward the navel. The average North American boy of today has well-developed pubic hair by the time he is 15. Axillary and facial hair begins to grow a little later, and few boys—whatever they may like to think—need to shave before they are 16 or 17. In addition, of course, puberty brings some growth of hair, increasing with age, on chest, shoulders, buttocks, arms, and legs.

With all this going on, even primitive people who have never heard of a hormone are perfectly able to mark, appreciate, and use in their customs,

Hercules slaying the Hydra, *a painting by 15th-century Florentine artist Antonio Pollaiuolo. Hercules, the classical archetype of the strong, he-man hero, wears a lion's head mane as a symbol of male strength and virility.*

magic, and folklore this clear and visible connection between body hair and sexual maturity. From the most ancient times, male facial and body hair has been seen as a symbol of virility. And in many cultures, by what psychologists would now term "displacement," the same role has been assigned, with no real biological justification, to the hair of the head.

By a natural extension, hair became also a symbol of fertility. Because its growth was associated with puberty it became the badge of the adult male's ability to procreate. Virility and fertility are, popularly if not medically, closely associated, and the seemingly almost magical power of hair to regenerate itself forged the hair-fertility link even more strongly. And so, from earliest times, hair has played an important part not only in puberty rites but also in ceremonies and rituals designed to propitiate the gods and to ensure fertility in humans, crops, or animals.

From all this there follows another simple equation: male hair equals virility, equals power, equals strength. It is a very ancient belief that a hairy man is a strong man. Perhaps it goes back to early man, whose epigamic hair won him sexual dominance. Certainly ancient writings and sculpture, as well as a great mass of myth and folklore from all over the world, show hair constantly fulfilling the dual role, symbolizing sometimes virility and sometimes physical strength.

The ancient Greeks were particularly keen on offering their hair to the gods, giving, as it were, some of their own fertility and strength in what they clearly hoped would be a two-way transaction. They sheared their hair and sprinkled it onto streams, to be carried by the water to fertilize the land and crops. At Delos and at Delphi, youths offered some of their hair, or their first beard, to the god Apollo, among whose many jobs was that of making the crops grow. Young men of Troezen might not marry until they had donated their hair or beard to the local deity Hippolytus.

Similar customs existed in Rome under the Empire. The historian Suetonius describes how the emperor Nero, after he had shaved for the first time, put the hairs in a pearl-studded gold box and dedicated them to Jupiter, in a typical blaze of publicity and to the accompaniment of a sacrifice of bullocks, at a gymnastic contest. The bullocks had to die, but Nero got away with a close shave. It seems likely, in fact, that hair was originally sacrificed as a convenient substitute for life itself. It had the obvious advantage of costing no blood or pain, and—unlike any other part of the body except the nails—it could regenerate itself. Because of this special property of renewal, together with its association with virility and fertility, it was a peculiarly appropriate substitute for, and symbol of, life and the life force.

Samson and Delilah, *by Dutch painter Anthony van Dyck (1599–1641). In the biblical story the cutting off of Samson's hair deprived him of his strength—an example of a man's head hair "displacing" his facial and body hair as a symbol of virility and power.*

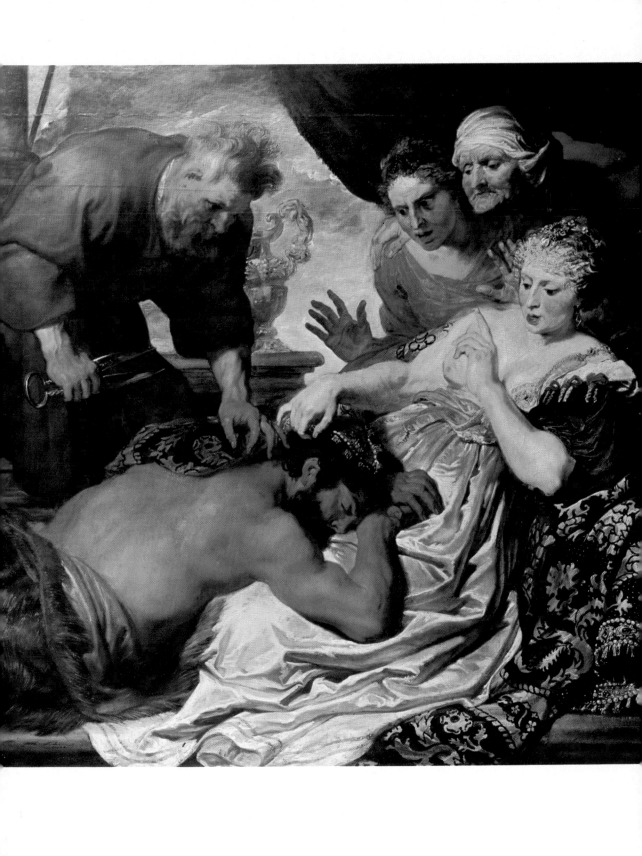

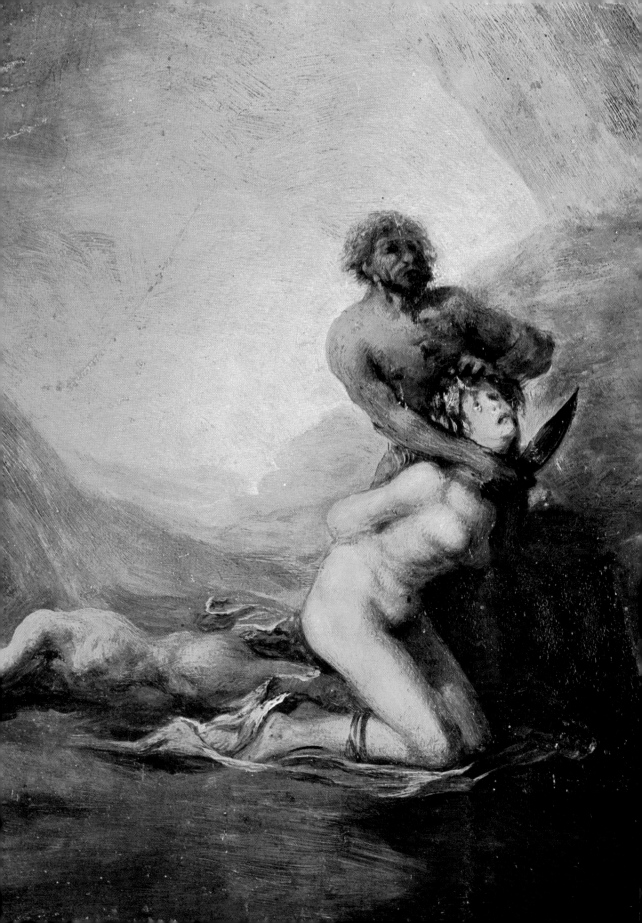

It almost seems that there could scarcely have been a hair left on a head in the ancient world. We read of Agamemnon, leader of the Greek army at the siege of Troy, tearing out handfuls of hair for Zeus; of Hercules sacrificing his locks on the tomb of his son Leucippus; and Achilles offering his at the funeral of his friend and comrade-in-arms Patroclus. The soldiers of an entire army, that of Pelopidas, the great general who freed Thebes from Spartan tyranny, clipped not only their own hair but that of their horses and mules to mark their leader's death in 364 B.C. Hair was offered in thanks for deliverance or in hope of deliverance, with always an appropriate and rapacious god to suit the cause. Mariners, of course, gave their salty locks to the sea gods—a custom depicted on a stone from Thessaly upon which are carved two plaits of hair dedicated to Poseidon, the Greek Neptune. One Latin poet, Lucilius, prudently hedging his bets, dedicated his hair to a long list of sea deities.

We have records of similar hair offerings from many places in the ancient world. It could be argued that a custom common to Greece, Rome, Egypt, Phoenicia, Arabia, and the Near East generally might well have spread from one country to another on the tide of war and trade. But the same emphasis on hair as a symbol of virility and strength is found in widely separated cultures in all parts of the world. The Old Testament story of Samson, who lost his strength when the treacherous Delilah had his hair cut off while he slept, has been absorbed into many cultures through Christianity, but, long before missionaries or modern mass media could reach them, the Masai of Kenya believed their chief would lose his power if his chin were shaved, and the Sioux Indians accepted hair so much as the seat of strength that they scalped their enemies to take away their power even in death.

This belief in a connection between hair and strength extended, of course, to the beard, often regarded as a sacred token of both strength and virility. Jewish Elders imposed a strict law forbidding the shaving of "the four corners of the face," which is still observed by strict Orthodox Jews. Some Jews exiled in clean-shaven societies have resorted to the drastic solution of removing chin hair with caustic paste rather than offend the letter of the law by using a razor. In ancient Babylon beards were held in such esteem that oaths were sworn upon them, and throughout history, in many cultures, to pull a man's beard was to assault his honor.

As a sign of manly strength—and to add to a fearsome appearance— beards and moustaches have gone to battle in a variety of shapes and forms. The ancient Britons, defying Caesar's armies, wore long, drooping moustaches dyed green and blue. The Black Prince, son of Edward III of

The whole nightmare world of hairy strength and bestiality, of women's ancestral fears of raping butchering hordes of savage invaders, is realized in this painting, The Decapitation *by Francisco de Goya (1746–1828).*

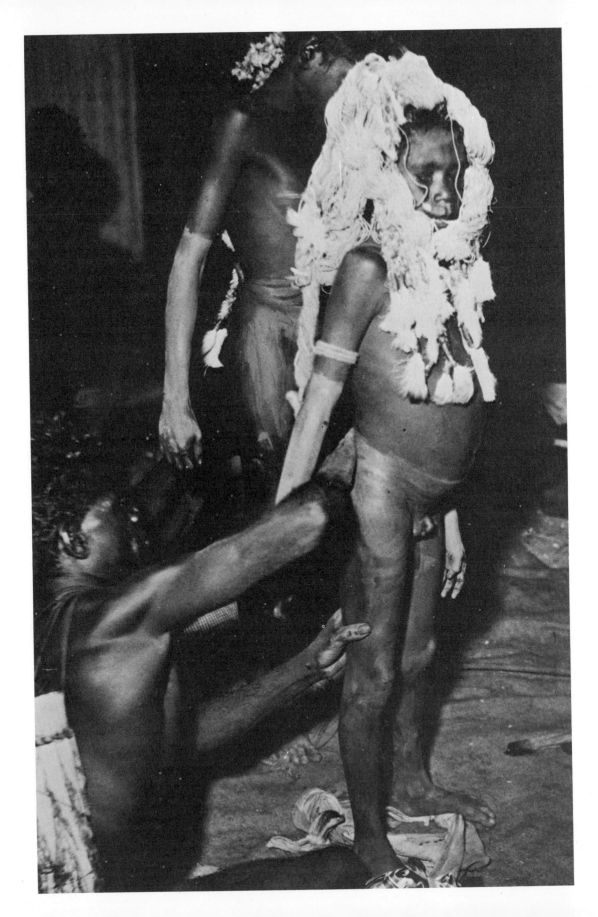

England and knightly hero of the 14th-century wars with France, is depicted with moustaches dangling somewhat incongruously outside his armor. Crusaders adopted Saracen moustaches, the Napoleonic wars favored sideburns, the Crimea allowed full beards to help also to keep the men warm. The American Civil War produced lushly bearded generals on both sides. World War I saw the thick, shaggy moustaches of the British infantryman and the waxed military points of officers. By World War II these had given way to the dashing whiskers sported by "Desert Rats" of the British 8th Army and pilots of the Royal Air Force.

The survival of such aggressive signals into modern warfare carries curious psychological implications. Long-range weapons, and the new strategy and mobility resulting from them, virtually eliminate the old face-to-face confrontation with an enemy. The instinct to flaunt defiant hair in war must now be more a matter of personal pride and satisfaction than of intimidation. The only time that the enemy is likely to see it is if he is your prisoner, or you are his or, worse still, dead. In the first two cases its intimidation value is unnecessary and in the last rather doubtful.

The truth seems to be that the moustache and beard of the fighting man have always had a three-fold motivation. The first is sexual invitation —a simple piece of strutting to attract the female. The second is the need for self-confidence: the soldier has to draw upon his courage and self-reliance, and there is no better way of buttressing both than by proclaiming his virility. The third is the aggressive instinct. This is the point made by Pearl Binder in her fascinating book *The Peacock's Tail* (1958). All male display signals, including hair, are like the gorgeous spread of the peacock's tail, and the peacock "is trying, not to attract a wife, but to frighten his enemy off his territory, and his gorgeous panoply is not a wedding garment, as Darwin was inclined to think, but a gladiator's vestment."

Perhaps in modern war only the first two motivations remain. But certainly, at least until very recent times, hair has always been a part of man's gladiatorial vestment and aggression display. The fierce, the frightening, or the abnormally strong throughout mythology have all been hairy. The biblical Samson, the Assyrian Gilgamesh, the Phoenician Melkarth, and the Greek Hercules, if not identical, are all emanations of the same hairy myth. All slew lions with their bare hands, all were men of prodigious strength, and all are represented in their different cultures in the same basic way, as powerful, hirsute, and bearded. Harald, the fierce Viking warrior who unified Norway in the 10th century, went down in history as Harald Fairhair, and among the chieftains of the Frankish tribes there was even one known as Clodion the Hirsute. The Frankish king Clovis, who

An Australian Aborigine boy being painted and decorated for the puberty rites that will mark his initiation into manhood. Because the growth of specifically male hair—that of the face, the chest, and the pubic region—is an obvious outward sign of puberty, hair plays a part in the puberty rites of many peoples. This boy, for example, wears a headdress that symbolizes an animal's mane or the lush hair and beard of early man—it represents male potency.

reigned between 481 and 511, describes how his people chose their kings from the hairiest of their warriors and adds that a king who failed in courage lost not only his throne but also his hair.

But if hairy strength and a certain nobility sometimes go together, so also does hairy strength and bestiality. It echoes in sinister whispers of werewolves, and in the dark, legendary horrors of rampaging hordes of berserkers and barbarians, not to mention the race that terrorized, ravaged, and raped its way through Europe, to be conquered in the end by Caesar and to be called by him the hairy Gaul.

Shaving the hair of a defeated enemy was a common humiliation, and one imposed by Rome on both the hairy Gaul and the almost equally hairy Briton, who, although beardless, wore long hair and long moustaches. Shaving of both beards and hair as a punishment has been popular in many cultures at many and varying periods. One poor Spartan, convicted of cowardice in war, was reputed to have been made to wear half a moustache. In his entertaining and informative book *Beards* (1950), Reginald Reynolds speculates on whether the wretched man had to grow his half moustache

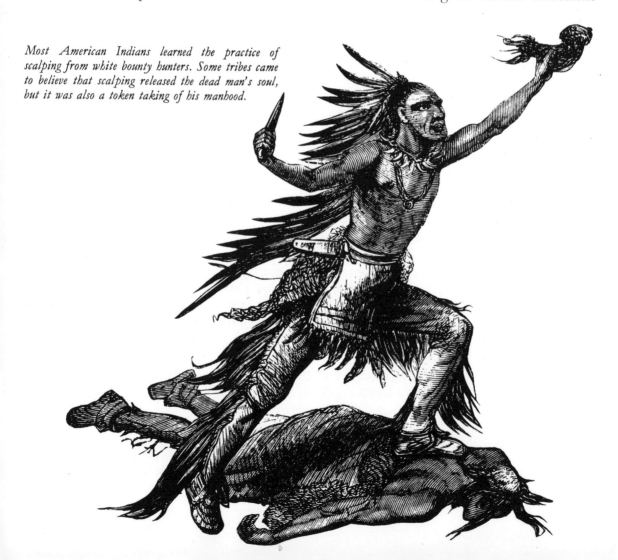

Most American Indians learned the practice of scalping from white bounty hunters. Some tribes came to believe that scalping released the dead man's soul, but it was also a token taking of his manhood.

especially, as it was normally a Spartan custom to keep the upper lip shaved. Punishment involving this forcible shaving or cropping has, of course, sexual implications. Because of the links between pubic hair and the genitals and, by "displacement," between head hair and sexual power, the cutting off of a man's hair is a symbolic castration. Hindu culture openly recognizes this and hair behavior and sex behavior are consciously associated. A Brahmin, for example, wears the tonsured tuft to represent sexual restraint, a shaven head for celibacy, or matted hair for total detachment from the sexual passions. In Buddhist Ceylon there is a similar distinction. Celibate monks have their heads shaved, to differentiate them from laymen leading normal sex lives, who wear their hair long. The Roman Catholic Church has a similar tradition for its monks, and even today young men embarking on training for the priesthood have a lock of hair cut off by the bishop, as a sign that they are turning away from the world. Except in some orders—such as the Franciscans, who by contrast *must* wear beards—or where special permission is granted, priests wear no facial hair, and this may be seen as a sign that they do not exercise their virility and are in that sense sexual non-combatants.

In *The Unconscious Significance of Hair* (1951), the psychiatrist Charles Berg suggested that in modern times the sexual symbolism of hair has been repressed into the unconscious under the veneer of civilization and the weight of cultural and social conventions. He quoted a mass of clinical evidence in support of this theory. Hair and the cutting or shaving of hair constantly turned up in his patients' dreams, and could be related under analysis to their sexual fears. Dr. Berg also argued that hair is an exhibitionist object: it is the only phallus that the conventions permit a man to show in public. It is this that underlies a man's pride in his hair and the time and effort he will spend on beautifying it. It also accounts for his anxiety to keep his hair groomed and under control. Untidy, up-standing hair is socially unacceptable—it represents the erect penis.

The idea of death, the loss of a loved person, as a castration or cutting off, fits neatly into the theory. Dr. Berg believed that this is why mourning is symbolized in so many cultures by shaving the head. He cited the Trobriand Islanders of the southwest Pacific as an example of this. He also saw their "Kayasa" ritual as a confirmation of the exhibitionist use of hair. This ceremony takes place after a long period with no deaths, when men have had a chance for their hair to grow long. The men assemble in a central place, dress their hair with long-pronged Melanesian combs, and display it to the women, who admire and pronounce judgment on its quality and beauty. Another example of the connection of hair with exhibitionism of sexual potency was seen by Dr. Berg in the custom once practiced in Uganda of a father of twins not cutting his hair, or cutting it in a special way, to distinguish him from ordinary, less virile men.

There seems little of the "unconscious" in this kind of display, or in the very explicit significance of the opposite display of shaved heads to denote celibacy that survives in some religious orders today. So, although Dr. Berg's arguments may hold good for his patients and perhaps for other inhibited or sexually repressed people, the great majority of us quite consciously accept the sexual significance of hair. Shakespeare had little doubt of it when writing for his Elizabethan audience, playing for a laugh through Sir Toby Belch's bawdy comment on Sir Andrew Aguecheek's hair: "It hangs like flax on a distaff; and I hope to see a housewife take thee between her legs and spin it off."

Certainly men's fear of losing their hair exists at a conscious level. Dr. Berg argued that "normal concern or anxiety about the hair becoming thin or falling out, alopecia, or becoming grey, are displacements of castration anxiety," but they are more likely to be simply a very natural concern for appearance, and a resistance to a sign of the aging process with its unwelcome reminder of inevitable mortality. It can be argued, of course, that, because baldness is so often part of old age, and old age brings failing sexual powers, the man noting the first hint of falling hair and a receding hairline feels himself moving into the cold shadow of impotence. In this sense perhaps Dr. Berg's castration complex is relevant, and undoubtedly some men do react in this way. Where they do, it is a

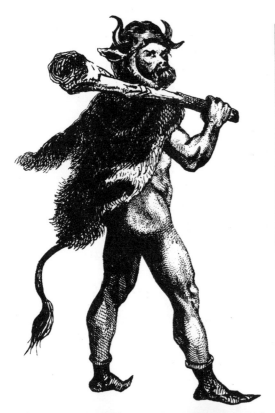

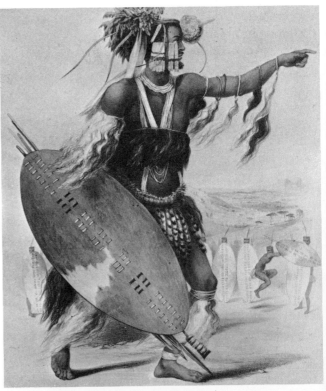

question of ignorance being not bliss but misery. For it is ignorance echoing ancestral fears that underlies this anxiety, and only the anxiety itself that can have any effect on virility by shattering the confidence essential to sexual success.

This is the only basis for the belief that baldness either affects virility or signifies lack of it. The truth is rather the opposite. For modern medical knowledge has established that most baldness, far from being due to some lack of masculinity, is due to an excess of it. It has now been proved that overproduction of male hormones (androgens) is a vital contributory factor in male pattern baldness.

Male pattern baldness is the name now commonly given to both early baldness (alopecia prematura) and baldness in old age (alopecia senilis), which together form over 95 per cent of all cases of baldness. It is estimated that about one man in five starts to go bald soon after adolescence and is very bald by the age of 30. Another one in five retains a fairly full head of hair until after the age of 60. The remaining three lose their hair more gradually, with the period of greatest loss coming after the age of 50.

Hippocrates, the father of medicine, observed that "eunuchs do not grow bald." Almost 25 centuries later, Dr. James B. Hamilton made a study in a Midwestern institution on a selected group of men who had been demasculinized in youth through accident or injury, or who for biological reasons had failed to mature sexually. He found not one case of baldness among them, not even a receding hairline. But when he administered male hormones to the subjects, some of them began to lose their hair. They were those from families in which baldness was common. No amount of hormones would produce baldness where no hereditary tendency existed.

And so it is not after all so simple. There is a double trigger mechanism at work. But do the sex hormones cause baldness only under the influence of heredity? Or does heredity result in baldness only when triggered by the sex hormones?

An American doctor, Armam Scheinfeld, has gone a long way toward providing an answer to these questions. He believes that there are specific genes for baldness, carried by both men and women. In a man only one set of genes is required to produce a proneness to baldness that may be triggered off by the male sex hormones. A woman must receive a set of these genes from both parents before she is likely to be affected, and even then she will suffer only partial baldness or thinning. This explains how the glandular makeup of the two sexes governs the way in which the baldness gene expresses itself. It explains Dr. Hamilton's results with his

A Germanic warrior of Europe's Dark Ages (far left), clad in an animal's skin, and a Zulu warrior of the 19th century (left), wearing strings of hair on his arms, legs, and body, are both using hair—animal or human—to make their appearance seem more terrifying. They are reverting to the epigamic hair of early man.

"eunuchs." It explains why women so rarely go bald. It explains why women suffering from a certain type of tumor on the adrenal gland, which results in a high production of male sex hormones, may suddenly go bald, and why, when the tumor is removed, both the baldness and other masculine characteristics (such as facial hair) disappear. It explains why, at the menopause, diminishing production of female hormones can so change a woman's hormonal balance that balding and coarse hair growth on the face may sometimes follow.

It is possible on the basis of hereditary tendency roughly to calculate the chances of baldness. Dr. Irwin Lubowe, a New York trichologist, has devised one simple method that recognizes only two very broad family categories. The first is the "positive" family, in which the men of over 60 and the women have good heads of hair. The other "negative" group takes in families in which some degree of baldness appears, the women having thin hair and the men being completely bald or having bald patches. It is enough to determine to which group parents and grand-parents belong, although by tracing still farther back more accurate predictions may be made. On this basis, if a man from a "negative" family marries a "negative" woman, their sons are faced with the near certainty of some degree of baldness. If a "negative" man marries a "positive" woman, the sons have only a 2 to 1 chance of baldness.

Another theory is that baldness is caused by impaired circulation in the scalp. This also would account for baldness running in families. Circulatory troubles may be related to the shape of the skull, which is an inherited characteristic. The "egghead," who is so often bald, fits neatly into this theory. His oval, egg-like skull makes it more difficult for the blood to circulate upward to the scalp. Other evidence in support of the circulation theory is provided by the usual pattern of male baldness. Hair is usually retained, even in fairly advanced baldness, at the sides and back of the head, where there are thin layers of muscle and fat. The temples, front, and top of the skull, devoid of muscle structure and with only a very thin fatty layer, go bald. Apparently, fat and muscle tissue protect against balding by cushioning the blood vessels and preventing vaso-constriction. The pressure of a tight scalp appears to reduce the fatty layers. When M. Wharton Young, an anatomist of Howard University, Washington, D.C., carried out experiments with monkeys in which he surgically tightened their scalps, he produced "persistent baldness closely resembling the human types."

If it is true that baldness is a result of bad circulation, it can be accounted for in evolutionary terms. Rival species had so much greater speed and

Opposite: the rugged, unshaven look of a modern male sex symbol—in this case Italian movie star Franco Nero. Overleaf: hair and the making of love.

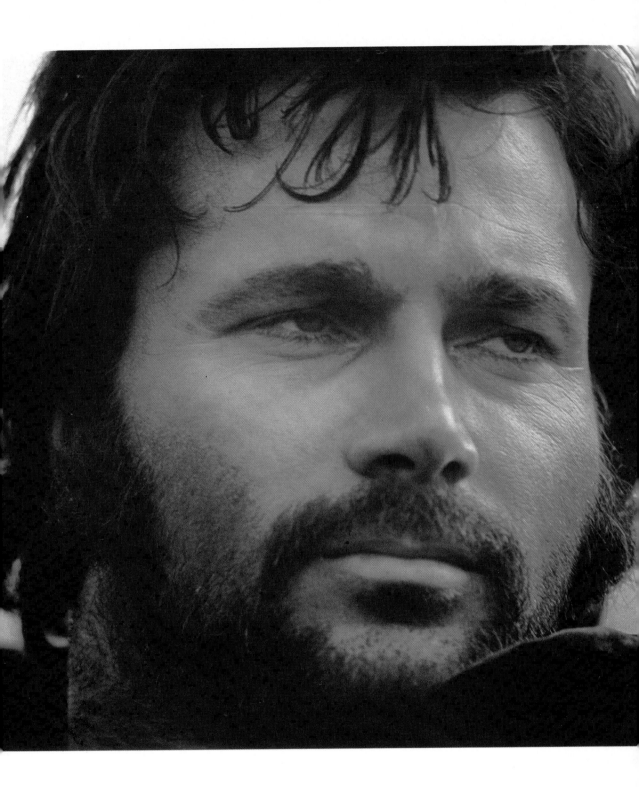

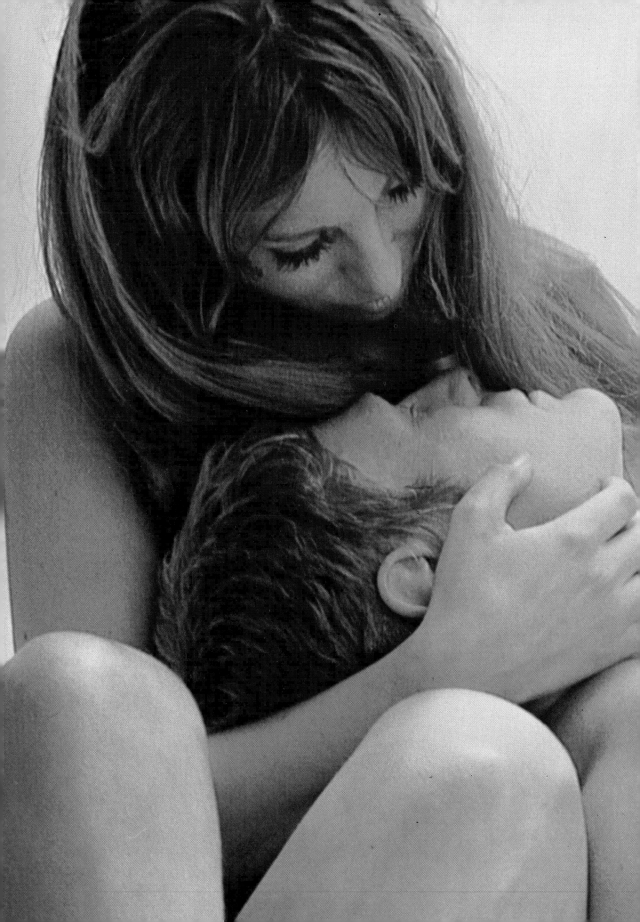

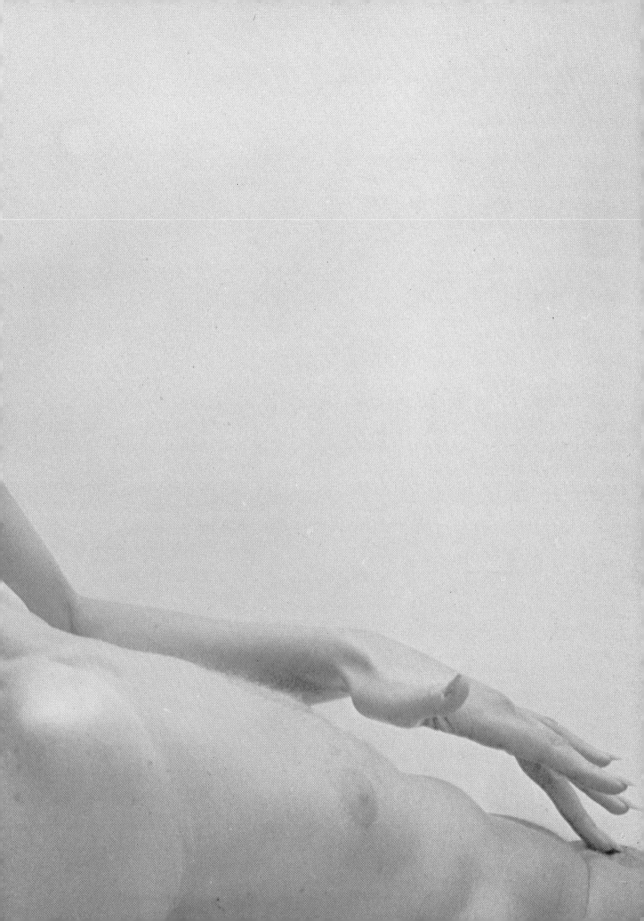

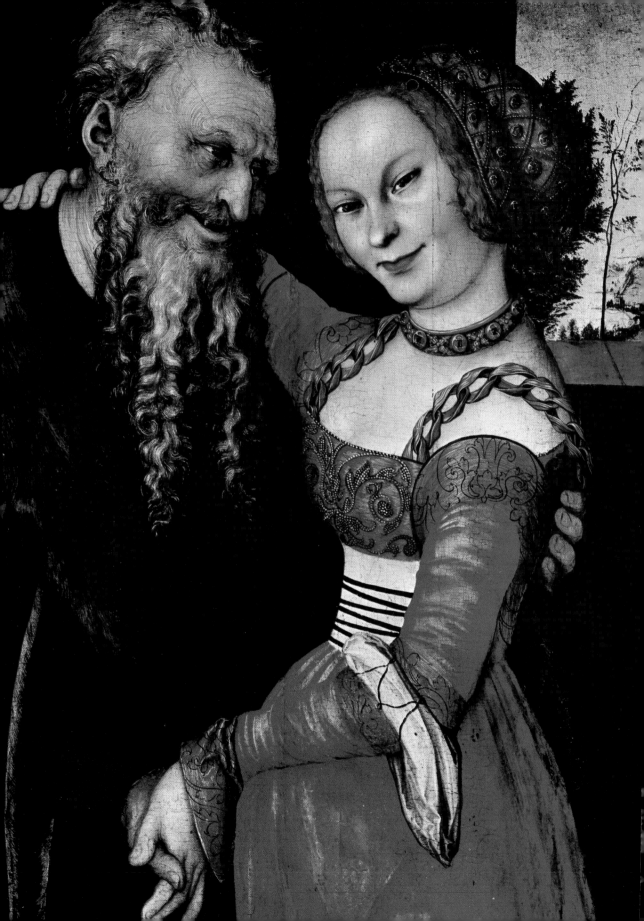

strength that man's survival depended upon him developing a more versatile and efficient brain than theirs to give him the cunning and ability to improvise and adapt in his dangerous and hostile world. We know that the size and weight of his brain gradually increased. Perhaps in some individuals skin growth did not match brain growth and the skin of the scalp became overstretched, reducing the circulation to the hair. Over generations this could have become a transmissible characteristic baldness. As we have seen, it is very difficult to dredge up any real evidence about hair before recorded history, but at least observation in the present gives this idea strong support. Baldness is rare in primates other than man.

But circulation can also be impaired by stress, anxiety, and emotion, and so another and very fashionable theory is that the tension of modern life plays a big part in what appears to be an increased incidence of baldness today. The fact that primitive races are usually exempt from baldness is offered in support of this idea, as is the increasing tendency to hair loss in women, who, happily emancipated, now bear their fair share of stresses.

Perhaps the most charming theory comes from two psychiatrists, Thomas A. Szasz and Alan M. Robertson of the University of Chicago, who tell us that laughter can make us bald. The facial nerve, which allows fluidity of facial expression, has branches that activate the muscles of the scalp and ears. Broad smiles and hearty laughter cause this muscle to pull on the scalp and tighten it, and, worse still, the suddenly tautened muscles themselves constrict the blood vessels supplying the hair.

Each theory, of course, suggests its own remedy, but possible cures for baldness are discussed in a later chapter. For the moment it is the possible causes that are important, in the bearing they may have on the widespread beliefs associating male baldness with sexual power or loss of power. It is true that certain types of hair loss can be due to poor general health or to specific diseases, such as syphilis, that clearly can affect virility. But, leaving aside emotional tension, which never did anyone's libido any good, the causes of normal male pattern baldness in early or middle life can have no adverse bearing on virility—except, perhaps, a psychological one. Loss of hair may bring loss of confidence, because of personal vanity and the need for reassurance through a young appearance, particularly in an age when youth is given so much status and adulation. It is a sad fact that men who feel that they are no longer attractive—and, above all, feel that it *matters* that they are no longer attractive—*become* less attractive. It is particularly foolish perhaps for men to worry in this way, because male beauty has never been given a high priority by women choosing either husbands or lovers.

In The Ill-matched Couple *by German painter Lucas Cranach the Elder (1472–1553), the old man, with his thinning, graying locks and straggly beard, lusts after the young woman. And she, for her part, finds an old man's gold more pleasing than a young man's golden hair.*

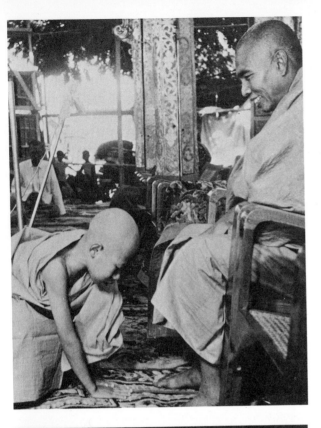
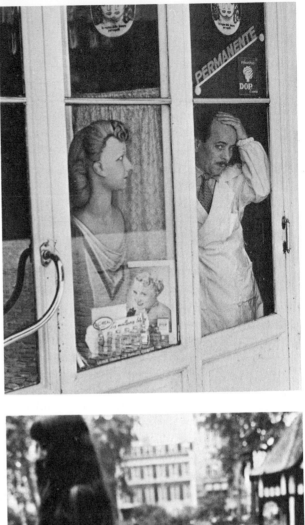
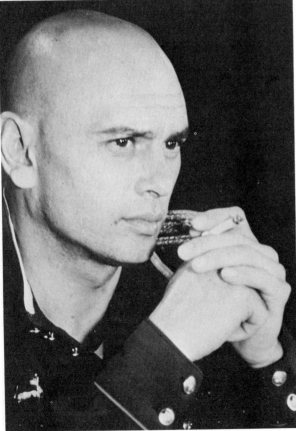
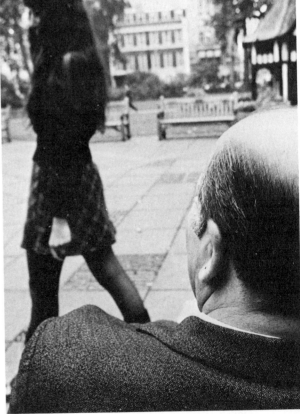

Some of the anxiety, of course, may be related to jobs and careers rather than to an imagined handicap in the sexual stakes, for in business too the emphasis is more and more on youth. Either way there can be serious consequences. Baldness may be a joke, useful for a laugh along with mothers-in-law in the after-dinner speech, or to portray the cuckold or the comic in a theatre, but to those men who fail to adjust to premature hair loss, it is no joke at all.

It is all the more sad and illogical when modern medical knowledge shows there to be no foundation for the bald man's worries, but suggests rather that he should wear his baldness proudly as almost a badge of virility. The same hormones that cause a man's facial and body hair to grow at puberty can cause his head hair to start receding shortly afterwards, if the hereditary tendency is present. The sex hormones that give the he-man his hairy chest can later doom him to a bald pate.

Some cultures have equated baldness with virility, or, at least, have not equated it with lack of virility. Suetonius quotes these ribald lines from verses sung by soldiers at a Triumph of Julius Caesar:

> On the girls of Gaul you made your splash,
> Hard-up you've come to raise more cash.
> Ho, watch your wives, you men of Rome,
> We bring the bald-head lecher home.

And yet it is said that, of all the honors he received, Julius Caesar prized the laurel wreath most, because it hid his baldness. So presumably even he minded about it, but not to the point of allowing it to sap his confidence. Easy enough, perhaps, for a man who could signify life or death merely by a gesture of his thumb. Great temporal power must make a man more sure of his power over women, whatever his physical short-comings. A throne, an empire, and a victorious army add up to about the ultimate in epigamic signals. Napoleon had all three, and clearly the fact that he began to go bald as early as 23 made no difference to his success in attracting women. And yet he, too, probably minded; there is a delightful anecdote, from the pen of his valet, describing how he once met the Czar Alexander of Russia to discuss the future of Europe and ended by discussing cures for baldness.

In contemporary terms, when a screen image can wield almost as much influence as an emperor once did, the film star Yul Brynner must have set the seal of sexual power and attraction firmly on bald heads. But still young pop idols toss long unruly locks and display bare hairy chests as they perform their sexual charades, perpetuating the other myth for which history finds just as many proofs. "Vir pilosus, seu fortis, seu

The male feeling that baldness is a humiliation is not a universal one. To the Burmese boy (top left) a bare, shaven head is the proud badge of his admission to a Buddhist monastery. Yul Brynner (bottom left) made a bald head a positive symbol of tough masculinity and his shaved head enhanced rather than diminished his appeal to women. But the hairdresser at his shop door (top right) is clearly worried; is it only professional anxiety, because his balding head is a bad advertisement? The businessman in a London square (bottom right) may or may not have his inhibitions, but at least his bald head does not stop him looking at the long-haired, mini-skirted girl.

libidinosus" was the Roman saying—"The hairy man is either strong or lustful." The belief was echoed by the pioneer of modern sexology, Havelock Ellis: "Of all physical traits vigour of the hairy system has most frequently perhaps been regarded as the index of vigorous sexuality. In this matter modern medical observations are at one with popular belief . . . ." Havelock Ellis was speaking, of course, of male facial and body hair, which, as we have seen, differs in structure, texture, purpose, and initial growth impetus from the hair of the head. But, despite his confident assertion, equating even this kind of hair with virility is extraordinarily difficult to substantiate. Men demasculinized before puberty usually grow only sparse body hair, but so do Negroes, who have a special reputation for virility. On the other hand an anthropologist, O. Ammon, took measurements of nearly 4000 French conscripts at the end of the last century and found that the hairier the man the greater his chest measurement and the greater the diameter of his testicles. But whether bigger testicles equal greater virility is, needless to say, undemonstrable.

It is difficult to assess even how women react to male body hair. Does it attract them? Do they believe the hairy lover is a virile lover? Men have written a great deal about women, describing their bodies in loving or lusting detail, but women have rarely written in the same way about men. This is not only because custom, and lack of education and opportunity, prevented it. Even today women writers, painters, and sculptors show little inclination to do homage to the male form as men do to the female.

The truth is that women are far less influenced by physical appearance than are men, and this is especially true in the erotic sense. The American sexologist Alfred C. Kinsey, in his statistical studies of human sexual behavior, found that 72 per cent of male subjects had an erotic response to the mere sight of women, clothed or unclothed, while only 58 per cent of the women reacted in this way to men. The contrast was even more marked when Kinsey showed his subjects nude photographs, drawings, and paintings of the opposite sex; only 12 per cent of the women showed any response, against 54 per cent of the men. But perhaps women are becoming less inhibited, or perhaps they require an emotional or sensual situation with which to identify, for it is reported that women in the audience have reacted strongly to the sight of male pubic hair in the film of D. H. Lawrence's novel *Women in Love,* although it is not clear whether their shrieks are of shock or excitement, or a mixture of both.

In an attempt to find out, among other things, contemporary female attitudes to male hair, a survey was carried out for this book by the Physician to a major British university. It must be stressed that the sample

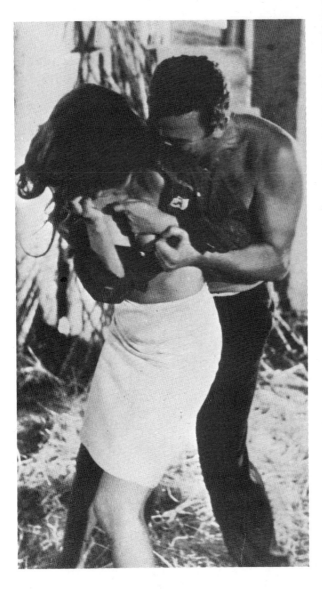

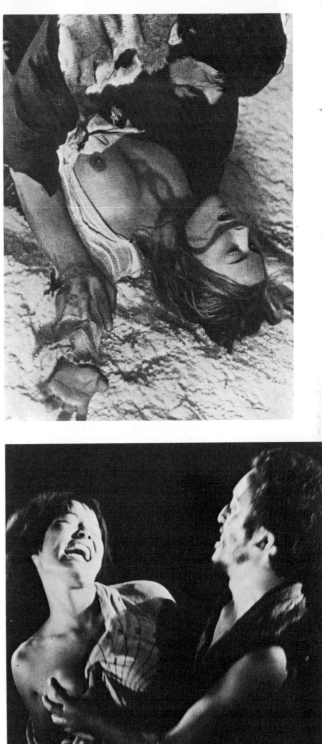

There is little evidence that hairy men are any more potent or virile than more sparsely covered ones, but popular belief still equates hairiness with maleness and motion-picture makers still use hairy chests, unkempt head hair, and unshaven faces as symbols of brute virility. These three scenes of rape—which is the ultimate expression of aggressive virility—are from the US film 10,000 Rifles (above), the Polish Muketa Iasatova (top right), and the Japanese Onibaba (right).

58

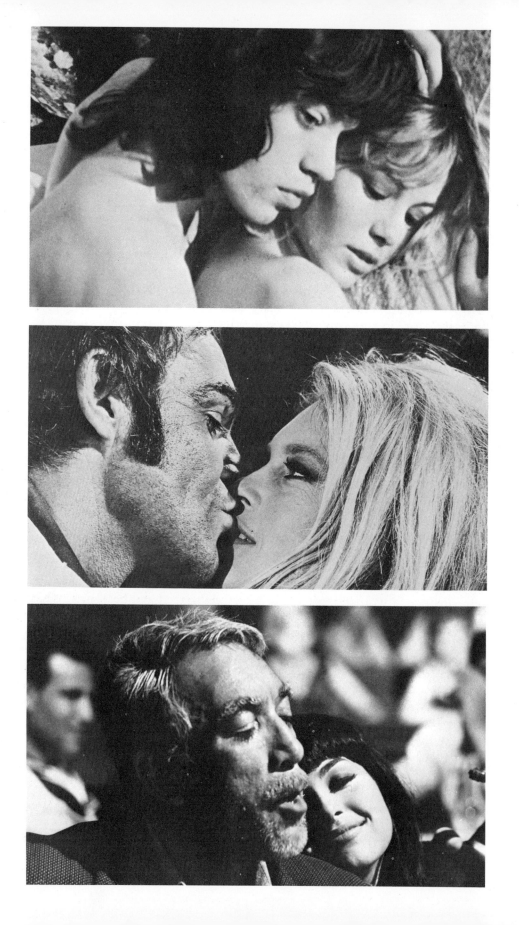

of some 200 men and women questioned in the survey is too small to offer more than a guide line. And it was not a completely random sample because all the subjects were attending the university health center, many for contraceptive advice, and almost all were sexually experienced. Eighty-seven per cent of them were under the age of 23, and all were under 35. Eighty per cent were English, the remaining 20 per cent belonging to 18 other nationalities.

The women were asked if they found male hairiness of chest, back, and limbs attractive. Ten per cent said they were actively "repelled" or "revolted" by it, and 28 per cent either that they were not attracted or not "particularly" attracted. Some 12 per cent—the "take-it-or-leave-it" brigade—found hairy men as attractive as non-hairy, and 25 per cent were attracted only provided the man was not *too* hairy—several of these said that they "couldn't stand hairy backs" and others were put off by "apes," "gorillas," or, in one case, "coconut mats." Of the remainder—roughly 25 per cent—two thirds were definitely attracted by male hair, one girl saying that she "liked a nice covering," and the rest very strongly attracted, some to the point of vaginally lubricating at the sight of a hairy man. Several said that a man could not be too hairy for them, and one wanted her men to be "like big bears."

The women's response to male pubic and axillary hair was also investigated. Almost half of them claimed that neither excited them, although some, on reflection, qualified their answer with some such phrase as "doesn't excite me *much*." Thirty-five per cent admitted that pubic hair excited them, several of them adding, rather enigmatically, that it made them "want to see more." Fourteen per cent found both pubic and axillary hair exciting. Two women expressed a particular aversion to axillary hair (thus neatly canceling out two who found it particularly arousing).

For a woman to be able to see and react to a man's pubic hair argues, in normal circumstances, a degree of intimacy. In public, and on first acquaintance, a woman must judge by a man's facial and head hair, which is all, in most societies, that she normally sees. How much importance does she attach to it? Even here literature is not very helpful. In considering hair and women's sex appeal, as we do in Chapters 3 and 8, there is almost an embarrassment of riches in poetry and in prose to illustrate how strongly men react to women's crowning glory. In the opposite direction there is almost nothing. Very few genuine female comments have come down to us. One of them was made by the first-century British queen Boadicea, who dubbed the Romans effeminate because they wore no hair on their cheeks and— perhaps worse—washed in hot water.

Until the 1960s the pure male hero of the cinema was almost always cleanshaven and well-groomed. With the coming of the anti-hero the image has changed—a rugged, careless, hairy look is in. Top, long-haired British pop-singer Mick Jagger makes love. Center, British movie star Sean Connery gives a bristly kiss to Brigitte Bardot. Bottom, US star Anthony Quinn, whose deliberately unshaven chin and cheeks contribute to his characterizations of rough, primitive lovers.

Most displays of more positive female appreciation have been penned by men, which means that they reveal not what women like but what men believe (or hope) they like. The Song of Solomon has a woman singing of her lover's charms:

My beloved is white and ruddy, the chiefest among ten thousand. His head is as the most fine gold, his locks are bushy, and black as a raven.

And, half a world away, a North American Indian song makes the woman describe her love in very similar terms: "hair flowing and dark as the blackbird that floats through the air."

Although the Anglo-Saxons, who put a price on everything, valued their beards so highly that they assessed the loss of a beard at 20 shillings, as against the breaking of a thigh at only 12, there is little evidence of women sharing quite the same enthusiasm. Shakespeare's contemporary, Ben Jonson, in his poem *Charis*, makes the woman of the title describe the man who would please her:

Young I'd have him too, and fair,
Yet a man; with crisped hair,
Cast in thousand snares and rings,
For Love's fingers, and his wings;
Chestnut colour, or more slack,
Gold, upon a ground of black,
Venus and Minerva's eyes,
For he must look wanton-wise.
Eyebrows bent, like Cupid's bow,
Front, an ample field of snow;
Even nose and cheek withal,
Smooth as is the billiard-ball;
Chin as woolly as the peach;
And his lip should kissing teach,
Till he cherished too much beard,
And made Love or me afeard. . . .

Clearly "woolly as a peach" is one thing, too much beard another, and Beatrice in *Much Ado About Nothing* is even more emphatic: Shakespeare makes her say, "I could not endure a husband with a beard on his face: I had rather lie in the woollen."

On the other hand, in one of the stories of the *Arabian Nights*, a girl argues that "a tree is only beautiful when it has leaves, and a cucumber only savoury when it is coarse and pimpled on the outside. Is there anything more ugly in the world than a man beardless and bald as an

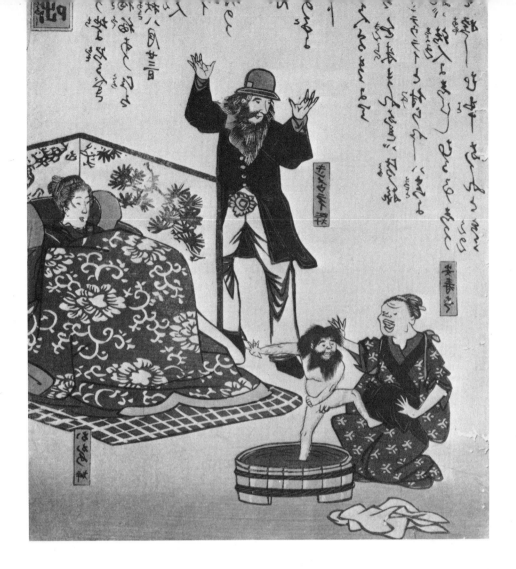

artichoke?" But she gives the game away later. She is thinking of beards as a proof of maturity and, although only 14, she does not like young lovers. "Do you think," she asks, "I would ever stretch myself out for love below a youth who, hardly mounted, thinks of dismounting; who, hardly stretched, thinks of relaxing; who, hardly knotted, thinks of unknotting; who, hardly arrived, thinks of going away; who, hardly stiffened, thinks of melting . . . and who, as soon as he has fired, thinks of retiring? Undeceive yourself, poor sister!"

What the girl said isn't evidence. Perhaps we should turn to history, which can certainly offer a fine selection of hairy male lovers, including Henry VIII of England, whose passions, not to mention his politics,

A 19th-century Japanese print (above) warns against the dangers of fraternization with white men. The inscription explains that the baby born to a Japanese girl and her sailor lover has white skin, is bearded and unnaturally hairy, can stand from the moment of birth, and is exceptionally strong. The cartoon plays upon the traditional Japanese abhorrence of body hair.

brought him six wives and more mistresses. The emperor Charlemagne, as well as a reputation for justice and nobility, had, and seems to have deserved, a reputation for virility and sexual appetite. He was described by a contemporary as tall, heavily built, and strong, with beautiful, well-combed, flowing hair, often scented "if the moment called for it." Presumably many moments did, for he had four wives and many mistresses, although chroniclers, perhaps prudently, name only five of them.

Henry VIII's royal contemporary, Francis I of France, has also come down through history as something of a sexual athlete. He was 23 when the two kings met for the jousting and junketings and devious diplomacy of the Field of the Cloth of Gold, and he was described as six feet tall (a great height for those days) and proportionately broad and robust, with a fresh complexion, dark hair, and a full beard, especially grown to enhance his regality. Pleasure-loving, skilled at sports and hunting, and never afraid of physical risk, Francis I embodied, as Charlemagne did, the vigorous, energetic, and aggressive male, but he also patronized the arts and found time for two wives and numerous mistresses. His first queen, Claude, bore him seven children in nine years.

Lord Byron, whose unconventional love affairs made him the romantic scandal of the 19th century, was another whose curly chestnut locks were admired not only by the ladies but obviously by himself too. He certainly wore curling papers in bed—presumably only when he was alone—and his long hair was to set the mode for Bohemian fashion.

Rasputin, the "mad monk" of Russia, was a hairy man able to exert the most extraordinary sexual power. Born to humble parents in a village in Siberia, he joined in 1904 a religious sect whose motto seems to have been "sin that you may be forgiven." Within a short time he had gathered around him adoring followers, whose wild dancing would end in a shameless orgy as Rasputin cried out the command "Try your flesh!" Despite this, or because of it, Rasputin ended up at the Russian court, where he continued to wield his power over the ladies, including the czarina herself. But there is a bizarre story, well-documented but understandably not included in the standard history books, which suggests that his strange power derived not so much from his hairiness as from warts on his penis, which gave the ladies especial and exquisite pleasure.

Other myths and legends are equally suspect, and many are contradictory. Men with red hair, men with dark hair, men with no hair, all in their turn are credited with superior virility. But truth is sometimes an elusive thing. Like beauty it may well lie in the eye of the beholder, and like faith it may in the end be only what we believe.

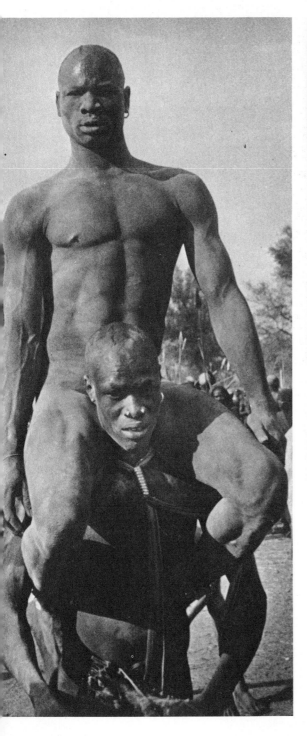

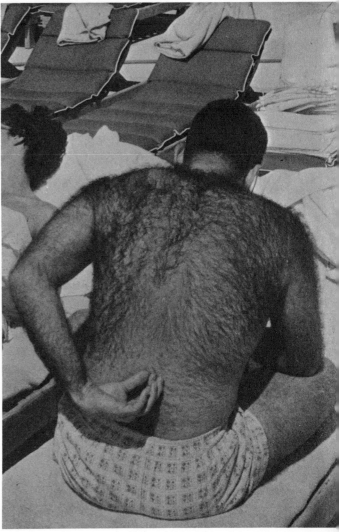

The popular belief that the hairy male is a virile male conflicts with another that credits the Negro with exceptional virility—for the Negro peoples generally have sparser body hair than the European. The muscular body of the champion Sudanese wrestler being chaired after a victory (left) is almost totally without hair. The white man sunbathing on the beach of a luxury resort (above) has a mat of hair on his back that would not disgrace a gorilla. Which is more exciting to women?

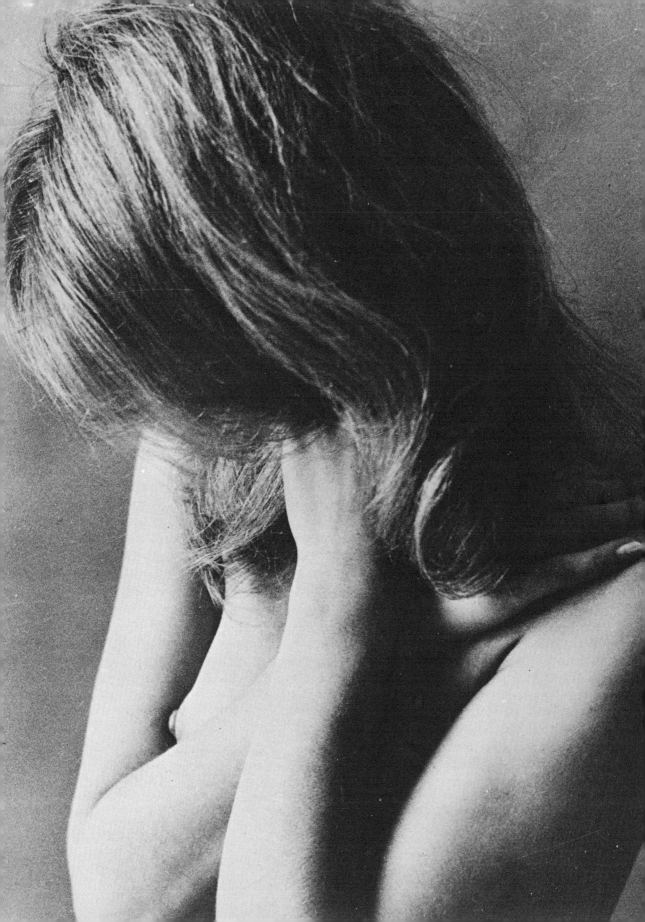

3 Hair and Female Sexuality

A woman's long hair, said St. Paul, "is a glory unto her." After the eyes, thought Havelock Ellis, a woman's hair is the first thing a man notices about her. "If you despoil the most startlingly beautiful woman of her hair," wrote the Roman satirist Apuleius, ". . . though she were Venus herself . . . she would not be able to seduce even her own husband." In other words, beautiful hair has always been a major item of a woman's sex appeal. Its color, its texture, its softness, its scent, are potent weapons in her sexual armory. Robert Burton, 17th-century author of the *Anatomy of Melancholy,* summed up its attraction: "In a word, the hairs are Cupid's nets, to catch all comers, a brushy wood, in which Cupid builds his nest, and under whose shadow all loves a thousand several ways sport themselves."

And yet, as we have seen, the hair of a woman's head differs so little from a man's that it is scientifically indistinguishable. Why, then, should it so attract the male? The answer seems to be first that, in Darwinian terms, the human female has become so denuded of hair on face and body that, by contrast, her remaining largest area of hair has gained in desirability, and secondly that, by "displacement," a woman's head hair is to the male a symbol of her pubic hair and hence of her very womanhood.

The pattern of a woman's *body* hair is, of course, very much a sexual characteristic, making its appearance at puberty. The sex hormones assert themselves earlier in girls than in boys, triggering growth of the first pubic hair soon after the breasts begin to develop, at about the age of 11. By the time the menstrual flow begins, this first hair has become wavy and fully pigmented, and the axillary hair has begun to appear. Finally, a light growth of hair develops on the arms and legs.

The erotic appeal of a woman's hair is a complex matter of texture, color, scent, and movement, but perhaps above all of the visual attraction of its soft flow against smooth skin. Men have always found loose, natural-looking hair sexier than the artificial creations of the hairdresser.

All this signals maturity and, specifically, the ability to bear children, so the link between hair and sexuality and fertility is even more direct than in men. So it is not surprising that in ancient Greece girls offered their hair at puberty alongside the boys in rites designed to promote fertility. Greek women also offered hair to Cybele for a happy marriage and to Athena on attaining it, and had to spare yet more locks in gratitude for the birth of a male child. One elderly prostitute, not to be outdone by virtuous wives, sacrificed a lock of her hair to Venus, perhaps in hope of retaining her beauty and prolonging her working life. The custom was not restricted to Greece. The Egyptian queen Berenice gave her hair for the safety in war of her brother-husband, Ptolemy; her shorn locks, it is said, were carried up into the heavens and became the constellation Coma Berenices.

The direct sexual symbolism of hair sacrifice was made explicit in the rites at the temple of Astarte, Phoenician goddess of fertility, at Byblus. The great anthropologist Sir James Frazer, in *The Golden Bough* (1890), wrote: "Here, at the annual mourning for the dead Adonis, the women had to shave their heads, and such of them as refused to do so were bound to prostitute themselves to strangers and to sacrifice to the goddess with the wages of their shame." According to Frazer, the goddess was prepared

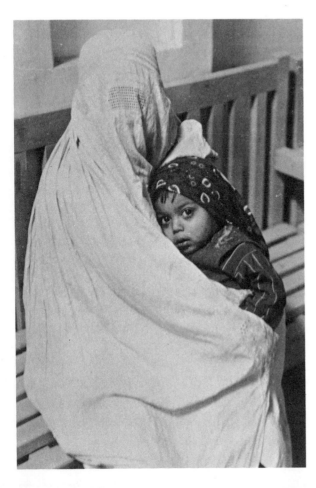

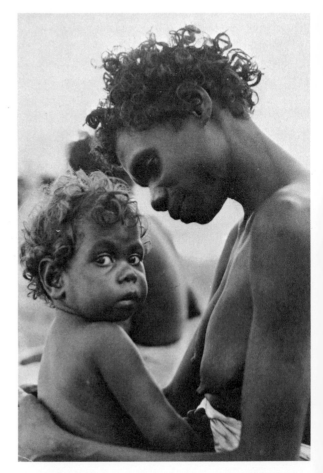

to accept the sacrifice of chastity as a substitute for the sacrifice of hair because both represented fertility. (We do not know what proportion of the women worshipers preferred losing their virtue to losing their hair.)

If surrender of hair can symbolize surrender of chastity, preservation of hair can equally symbolize preservation of virginity. There are many examples of this in the puberty rites of primitive societies. For example, girls of the Wafiomi tribe of East Africa, upon reaching puberty, were segregated from the rest of the tribe for a whole year, and during that time forbidden to cut their hair. A logical extension of the same symbolism is the cutting of girls' hair at or just prior to marriage, which is a recurring theme in the customs of many peoples. In Mecca, the hairdresser would cut off a bride's hair just above the forehead, arranging what was left in eight braids, and would also shorten her eyebrows. A very similar practice existed among the Bedouin in Iraq and in the Negev. Native Jewish women of Palestine often had both their hair and their eyebrows shaved off before marriage. Even today some Orthodox Jewish women crop their hair at marriage and afterwards conceal their natural hair from the sight of everyone except their husbands by wearing the *sheitel,* which nowadays is likely to be a perfectly ordinary wig.

Concealment is often a substitute for cutting off the hair. Roman Catholic nuns, who are married only to Christ, cover their hair with a coif. The Arabs long considered it more shameful for a married woman to be seen with her hair uncovered than to be seen naked. According to a mid-19th-century writer, Alexander Walker, in his book *Beauty:* "Among old-fashioned people, of whom a good example may be found in old country people of the middle class in England, it is indecent to be seen with the head unclothed; such a woman is terrified at the chance of being seen in that condition, and if intruded on at that time, she shrieks with terror, and flies to conceal herself." The obverse side of the same coin appeared in ancient Israel, where the woman suspected of adultery was made to wear her hair uncovered to indicate her disgrace.

In all this there seem to be two conflicting strands of hair symbolism. Loose, uncut hair is seen both as a symbol of virginity and as a symbol of promiscuity. Both aspects have retained their force into modern times. The girl in Edwardian England who put up her hair to signify that she had reached maturity was symbolically offering her virginity in the marriage market. On the other hand, when, in liberated France toward the end of World War II, women suspected of having consorted with the occupying German troops had their heads publicly shaved, it was the loose hair of promiscuity that was removed. There was also in this punishment a

Two mother and child scenes show two opposing attitudes toward the parts of the body a woman is permitted to display. The Moslem woman from Afghanistan (far left) is completely covered by traditional veils—even her face and hair must be concealed. But custom allows the African woman (left) to reveal not only her face and hair but also her breasts.

clear element of sadism, both directly, in the imposing of public humiliation, and indirectly, in that the head-shaving was a substitute for rape.

In other words, that particular punishment was probably more directly sexual than symbolically sexual. And modern man, who has fallen out of the habit of thinking in symbolic terms, will certainly find it easier to appreciate the erotic appeal of a woman's hair than to understand its symbolic meaning. Here he is at one with primitive peoples. Mutual grooming of the hair by men and women as a preliminary to intercourse is widespread among primitive tribes who have been examined by anthropologists, including the Dobu of the western Pacific, the Plains Indians of North America, and the Trobriand Islanders. In fact it is so widespread that it is tempting to see it as a survival of primate life, akin to the grooming behavior of the apes. Generally, hair has a more important role in the love play of primitive peoples than in that of more advanced peoples. The great pioneer anthropologist Bronislaw Malinowski, in *The Sexual Life of Savages* (1929), described the large part it played in the love-making of the Trobriand Islanders: "The lovers plunge their hands into the thick mop of each other's hair and tease it or even tear it. In the formulae of love-magic, which ... abound in over-graphic exaggeration, the expressions, 'drink my blood' and 'pull out my hair' are frequently used."

Whether it is a survival from our ape-like ancestors or, as Darwin thought, an evolutionary innovation, the erotic appeal of women's hair is immensely strong. It runs like a fascinating and sometimes fatal thread through mythology and history, poetry and prose. While the appeal of women's body hair is, as we shall see, often a question of cultural preference or of individual taste, that of head hair is almost universal. Almost everywhere in the world women's hair has been an object of sexual attraction. Its seductive power has gone into mythology with the story of the Lorelei, who sang on a rock overlooking the Rhine combing her long golden tresses, luring to their deaths unwise boatmen who raised their eyes. Legends of beautiful mermaids, common to many countries and many ages, echo the same irresistible and fatal power of flowing hair.

It is strange, therefore, that women, obviously aware of the effect their natural hair could have, and usually only too ready to exercise sexual attraction, should at certain periods of history have adopted deliberately outrageous and extravagant coiffures—often so expensively and elaborately contrived that they had to last, untouched, for weeks. A reasonable amount of styling and order in the hair could perhaps entice a lover, offering a challenge to convert cool sophistication into something less poised and perfect, but many of the towering edifices women have worn must have

Opposite: René Magritte's painting The Rape *(1934), in which a woman's body becomes her face, exploits the fact that head and body hair are prime attributes of female sexuality. Overleaf: Austrian painter Gustave Klimt (1862–1918) uses the flow of hair, echoed by the flow of gold, to emphasize the sexuality of his Danaë, the mistress of Zeus. On page 71: red hair has always had sex appeal. Top left, one of the numerous shades that can be achieved through modern hair tints; bottom left, a red-haired Venus by Lucas Cranach the Elder (1472–1553); bottom right, an auburn Saint Mary Magdalen by Titian (c. 1487–1576); top right,* Young Woman with Red Hair, *by 19th-century Italian Impressionist Frederigho zan Domenighi.*

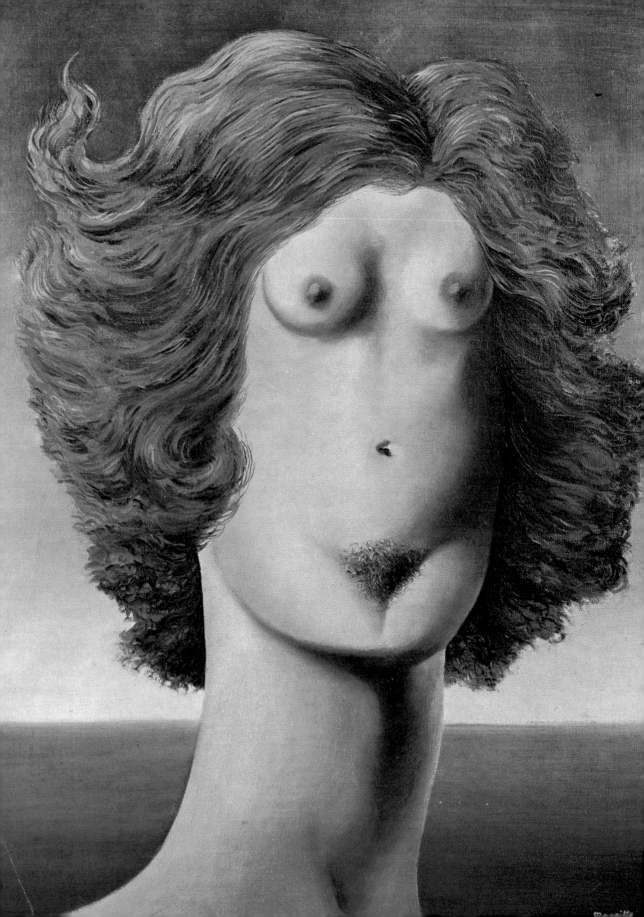

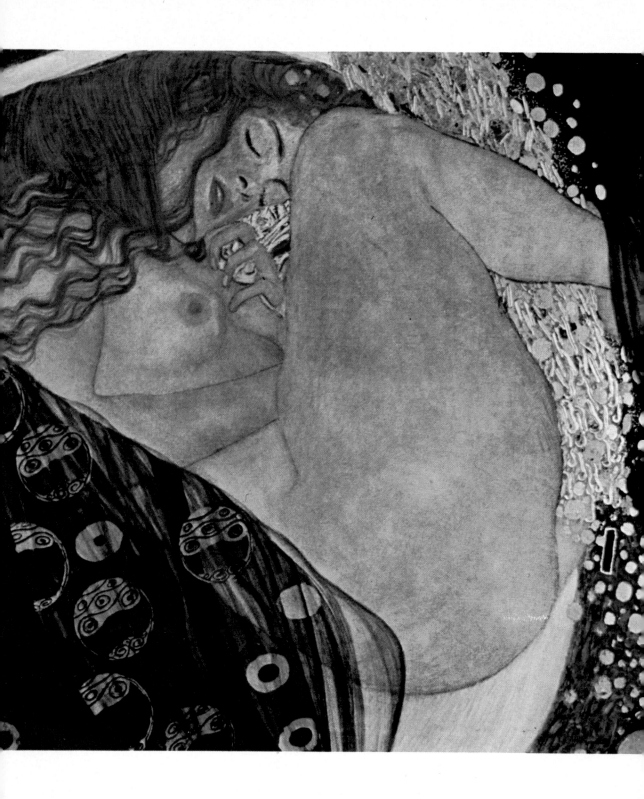

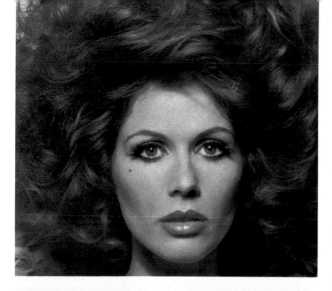

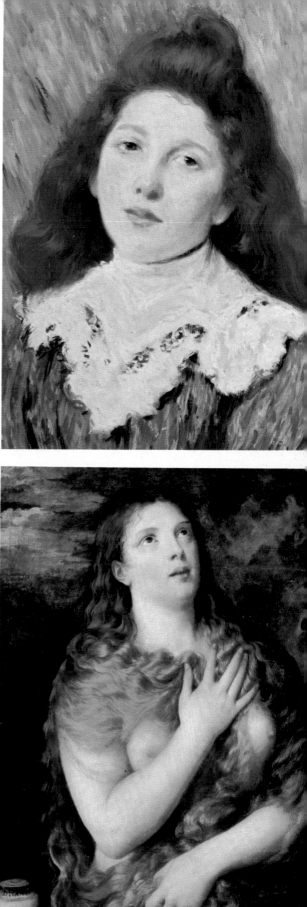

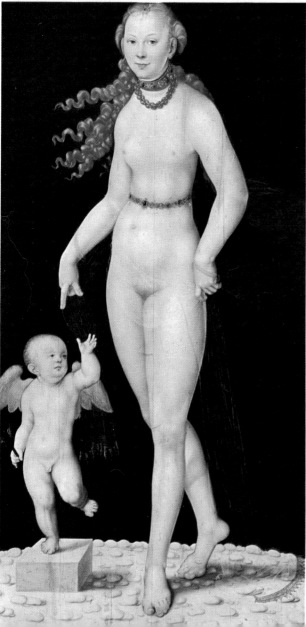

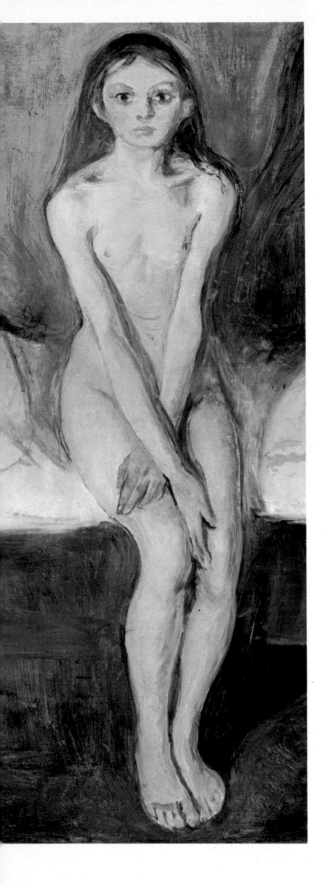
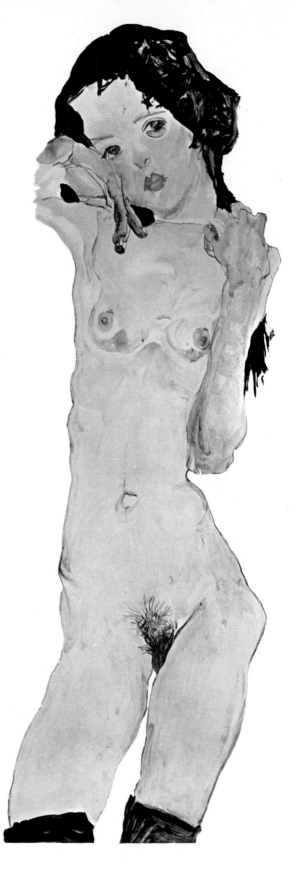

struck terror into the heart of the most ardent man, only too aware that the first hint of passion would bring the lot tumbling down, not in glorious disarray but strewn and scattered like a haystack. Highborn Japanese ladies, to avoid disarranging this kind of monumental hair style, often chose to sleep with their heads on a wooden or porcelain *k'ang,* and packed their husbands off to console themselves with geishas.

It is small wonder that the great Italian statesman and writer Baldassare Castiglione, laying down rules for Renaissance women in the early 16th century, advised them: "How much more doth a man delite in one, with her hair by happe out of order and ruffled," and a modern French sexologist, Georges Valensin, in *La Science de l'Amour,* has stated uncompromisingly: "It has been found that too majestic or too well arranged hair lacks erotic appeal; it should be left to hang loose in the sexual act and constraint is quite unsuitable." Perhaps this is because men equate looseness of hair with sexual looseness, or perhaps it is an expression of the male fantasy of the virile, aggressive caveman who seizes his woman by her long hair. Certainly men have urged women to set their hair free right through the ages. The English Cavalier poet Robert Herrick appealed to his lover Julia, whose hair was bundled up in a golden net:

Tell me, what needs those rich deceits,
Those golden Toyles, and Trammel-nets,
To take thine haires when they are knowne
Already tame, and all thine oune?
'Tis I am wild, and more than haires
Deserve these Meshes and those snares.
Set free thy Tresses, let them flow
As aires doe breathe, or winds doe blow. . .

But women always seem to have paid more attention to the demands of fashion than to the desires of men, and men have been oddly submissive to women's whims. In *The Conquest of Baldness* (1961), Gilles Lambert, it is true, tells a cautionary tale of one man who struck back. He describes how in Paris "quite recently" a Corsican petty government official was arrested for the murder of his wife. The only explanation he could give was: "She had cut off her hair to be in the fashion." More typical were the men of ancient Rome, who learned to accept philosophically the changing hair styles of their women—as many styles, according to Ovid, as there were honeybees in Hybla and wild animals in the Alps.

It was a Roman—Apuleius again—who wrote perhaps the most charming tribute ever paid to woman's hair: "What joy it is to see hair of a beautiful color caught in the full rays of the sun, or shining with a milder lustre and

Far left: Puberty, by Norwegian artist Edvard Munch (1863–1944). Left, nude girl by Austrian Expressionist painter Egon Schiele (1890–1918). One of the most obvious signs of puberty is the development of the typical mature female patterns of hair distribution.

constantly varying its shade as the light shifts. Golden at one moment, at the next honey-colored; or black as a raven's wing, but suddenly taking on the pale bluish tints of a dove's neck-feathers. Give it a gloss with spikenard lotion, part it neatly with a finely toothed comb, catch it up with a ribbon behind—and the lover will make it a sort of mirror to reflect his own delighted looks. And oh, when hair is bunched up in a thick luxurious mass on a woman's head or, better still, allowed to flow rippling down her neck in profuse curls! I must content myself by saying baldly that such is the glory of a woman's hair that though she may be wearing the most exquisite clothes and the most expensive jewellery in existence, with everything else in keeping, she cannot look even moderately well dressed unless she has done her hair in proper style."

Just as fashions in length and style change in different places and different periods, so do fashions in color. Red hair in particular has blazed an erratic trail. It has held its popularity in Italy and Greece right to this

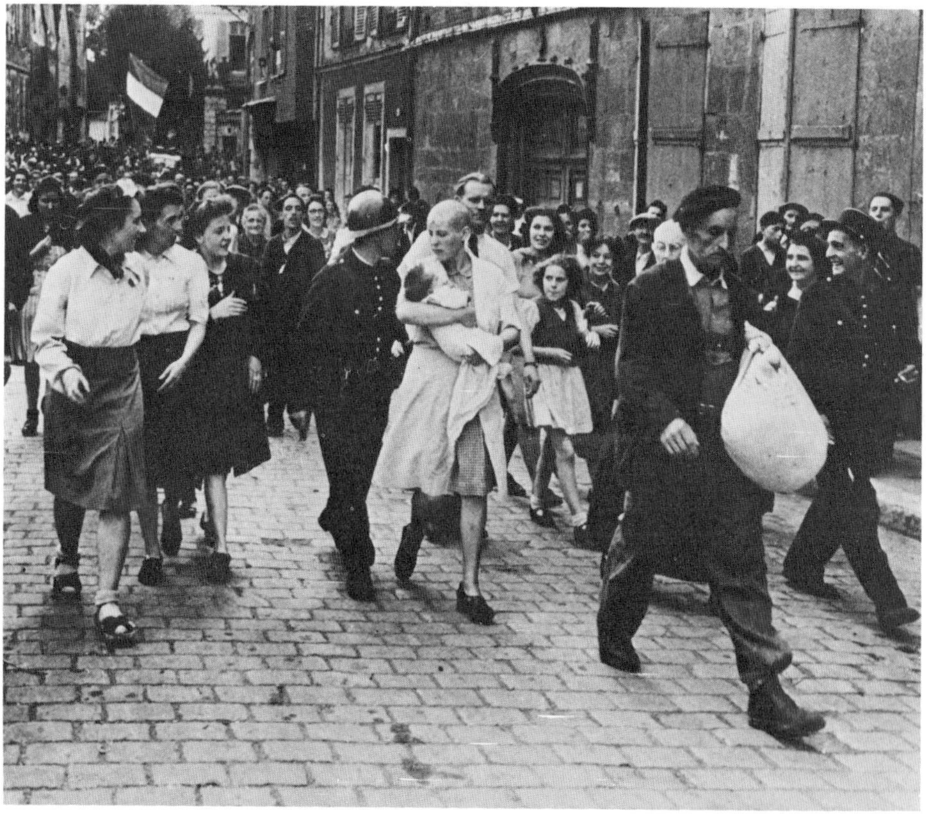

Paris, 1944. A mocking, hostile crowd surrounds a woman whose head has been shaved—the punishment imposed after the Liberation on many Frenchwomen suspected of fraternizing with the German occupying troops. The punishment has a symbolic significance as well as undertones of sadism.

day. When nature did not oblige, artifice had to. The glorious red-gold tone immortalized by the painter Titian in the hair of his Venetian women was usually achieved by sponging the hair with a solution of soda, alum, and black sulfur, and then allowing it to dry in the sun, spread out over the broad brim of a crownless hat. In England under Queen Elizabeth I, sandy-red hair became fashionable for a time, because the queen herself was red-haired when young. Nell Gwynne, the mistress of Charles II, was also a redhead. But at times in England, France, Germany, Spain, and America, red hair has been unpopular and distrusted. At the height of Europe's witch hunts, in the 16th and 17th centuries, many women suffered the shame and pain of being stripped, shaved, and "pricked" by a witch-hunter, endured torture, and were put to death, simply because they were redheads—and, preferably, young and attractive. The fear of red hair may have stemmed from the belief that Judas, who betrayed Christ, was red-haired. The 17th-century French scholar Jean-Baptist Thiers in his *Histoire des Perruques* gives this prejudice as one reason for wearing a wig: "Redheads should wear wigs to hide the color of their hair, of which everybody stands in horror because Judas, it is said, was red-haired." Shakespeare was obviously familiar with the same prejudice in his day, for in *As You Like It* he made Rosalind, speaking of Orlando, say, "His very hair is of the dissembling color," and Celia replies, "Something browner than Judas's." In Germany, barbers advertised all sorts of concoctions for altering the red shade of hair, and in America a newspaper was once driven to explain that 21 men in Cincinnati, who had married red-haired women, were color-blind and had mistaken red for black.

But the prejudice extends beyond Christian cultures—at one time Brahmins were forbidden to marry red-haired women. So Judas cannot bear all the blame. More probably the comparative rarity of red hair has made it suspect because unusual. In this century red hair has, in most of Europe and in the United States, come back into favor. Perhaps the legend that red-haired women are especially passionate has something to do with it, in an age when women are once again credited with sexual feeling. Equally, perhaps, effective semipermanent rinses have played a part, and the advent of color movies and color television has favored both redheads and blondes.

Fair hair has constantly held its place in the European ideal of feminine beauty. For long periods the woman with blonde hair has been the object of the European male's desire. A German gynecologist, Carl Heinrich Stratz, writing in 1899, thought that this was because fair hair harmonized better with the soft outline of a women's body. He believed that a woman's armpit hair should also be light-colored, but that her pubic hair should be dark "to emphasize the width of the pelvis and the obtuse angle between the *mons veneris* and the thighs," and that her eyebrows and eyelashes should also be dark to make the eyes look bigger.

Whatever the reason, fair hair has always had a very special attraction for men. The German poet Goethe warned against its power:

Beware of her fair hair for she excels
All women in the magic of her locks;
And when she winds them round a young man's neck
She will not ever let him free again.

The Lorelei and mermaids, so fatal to men, had long fair hair. So, often, had the dream princesses of the fairy tales, including the fatal Zoulvisia who let down her long hair, which was "like liquid gold," and drew up her suitor to the summit of her crystal tower. In *The Unconscious Significance of Hair,* Dr. Berg interprets this story in analyst's terms. The letting down of the princess's hair he relates to hair-exhibitionism and to the ability of a sexy woman to overcome the inhibitions that cause impotence in the man. He sees the suitor's entrance into the tower as a representation of the sexual act, and certainly Zoulvisia's first words to her suitor—"You have conquered me"—give some credence to his interpretation.

But fair hair, of course, symbolizes not just power but purity as well. The aesthetic quality of fair hair as something shining and pure like a flame, or precious like gold, would be enough to account for this to most people, but Dr. Berg relates it to the fact that fine, fair hair is less nearly related to pubic hair than any other, and so is further removed from any sexual association. It seems a shaky argument in view of the strong sexual attraction blonde hair has always exerted. The purity legend is perpetuated more by default, as it were, with warnings such as the proverb, "All are not maidens that wear fair hair," and the American poet Henry Wadsworth Longfellow's lines:

Often treachery lies
Underneath the fairest hair.

It is possible to argue that purity implies innocence, innocence may mean ignorance, and ignorance denotes stupidity. This extension of the old tradition could explain that 20th-century phenomenon, the dumb blonde. But such glib reasoning takes no account of the fact that the dumb blonde is often also the sexy blonde, whom gentlemen were once supposed to prefer. It seems more likely that the dumb-blonde image was a spinoff from the frenetic post-World War I period, when the most frivolous of the flappers were also the most likely to experiment with the new platinum-blonde bleaches. The image has survived yet another war and on through Marilyn Monroe (who once said, "I like to feel blonde all over") and Jayne Mansfield to the most recent and dumbest blonde of all, Goldie Hawn. But if the dumbness was allowed to dominate the sexiness in some blondes, there is very little dumbness and a lot of sex in such stars as Mae West, Marlene Dietrich, and Brigitte Bardot. They may seem strange descendants of the Lorelei, the mermaids, or the fairy-tale princesses, but these modern sex symbols rely just as much on the appeal of their blonde hair. Significantly, when Jean Harlow, platinum-blonde star of the 1930s, made a desperate protest against being exploited as a sex symbol by her studio, she did so by hacking off the blonde hair that had been made the trademark of her sex appeal.

Perhaps because blondeness can so easily be the product of a bottle of bleach, blondes have a reputation for being natural deceivers. Brunettes are supposed to have franker, more honest natures. A psychologist quoted by the London *Daily Mail* in November 1969 said: "If a man is serious about a girl he wants her to be natural. Anything artificial does not appeal to a serious thinking man who values quality. Generally speaking a man prefers a blonde for a mistress and a brunette for a wife. Brunettes have more integrity." If this makes the brunette sound dull compared with the blonde, it is only necessary to recall some of the sex symbols of their day who have gloried in their darkness—such as Hedy Lamarr, Jane Russell, Ava Gardner, Gina Lollobrigida, Elizabeth Taylor, and Claudia Cardinale. The true vamp is always dark-haired, perhaps because the contrast of dark hair with pale skin gives the brunette a more sexually dramatic coloring than the blonde.

But today hair colorants are so widely used, and so difficult to detect, that men would be foolish to jump to conclusions about a woman's character on the evidence of her hair color. Perhaps they should try out the strange theory of the Frenchman Augustin Galopin, whose book *Le Parfum de la Femme* was published in Paris in 1886. According to Galopin, redheads have the strongest scent of all women, brunettes are next, and blondes the most faintly scented. Redheads, and women with chestnut hair, smell of amber or of violets; brunettes have the scent of ebony; blondes have a much more subtle odor of amber or violets.

The belief that hairiness indicates virility in men is paralleled by one that hairiness indicates wantonness in women. Giovanni Battista della Porta, the great 16th-century physiognomist, thought that the thicker the hair the more wanton the woman. A 19th-century French doctor, Félix-Alexandre Roubaud, in his book *Traité de l'Impuissance,* made the same point more

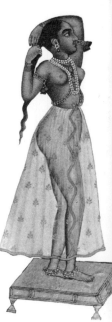

An 18th-century Indian miniature of a courtesan arranging her hair.

negatively. He wrote: "In the cold woman the pilous system is remarkable for the languor of its vitality; the hairs are fair, delicate, scarce and smooth, while in ardent natures there are little curly tufts about the temples." He was supported by his contemporary and fellow-doctor, Auguste-Ambroise Tardieu, who described the typical highly erotic woman as very hairy. The bawdy Abbé de Brantôme, in his *Les vies des dames galantes,* published in 1665 after his death, quoted a saying that hairy women are either rich or wanton, and claimed to know a great lady who was both.

Authentic records are (not unnaturally) hard to come by, but in 1894 a Danish researcher, R. Bergh, published a solemn report on 2200 young Danish prostitutes and noted an unusual amount of pubic hair on many of them, including those reputed to be the most highly sexed. Much the same results were reported by an Italian, Giovanni Battista Moraglia, who three years later made a similar study comparing prostitutes with other women, and came to the conclusion that both very thick body hair and a more than usual amount of down on the face were indicators of sexuality. Another Italian, Cesar Lombroso, reported in his book *Donna Delinquente* (1895) his own findings that prostitutes generally tended to be hairy.

Unfortunately none of this is of much help to the hopeful male, who may be badly mistaken in assessing sexual potential if he makes any assumptions based on a glorious mass of head hair. Havelock Ellis makes this clear. "In abundance the pubic hair corresponds with the axillary hair; when one region is defective in hair the other is usually so also . . . . But the hair of the head usually varies independently . . . ." With axillary hair so often shaved, and with the conventions of normal civilized clothing fashions concealing so much, what can a man do? Havelock Ellis offers one clue: "Strong eyebrows," he advises, "usually indicate a strong development of pubic hair."

In any case, hairiness is an unreliable guide to female sexuality. The Mediterranean races, who certainly carry more body hair than most others, have always had a reputation as passionate lovers, but psychological factors are so closely involved in women's sexual response that any such generalization as this is wildly dangerous. Modern endocrine knowledge offers little factual evidence either way, although an over-secretion of androgens (the male hormones), which produces a male-like hair distribution in women, has been linked with enhanced sexual feeling. Ignorant or unscrupulous men have, in fact, been known to feed androgens to young women for their aphrodisiac effect. The results have often been tragic, as well as self-defeating; the side effects include ugly facial hair growth and a croaky, masculine voice.

Blonde sex symbols of the cinema. French star Brigitte Bardot (top left) had a long line of predecessors that stretched back through America's Marilyn Monroe (top right) and Britain's Diana Dors (bottom right) to the star who began it all, Jean Harlow (bottom left).

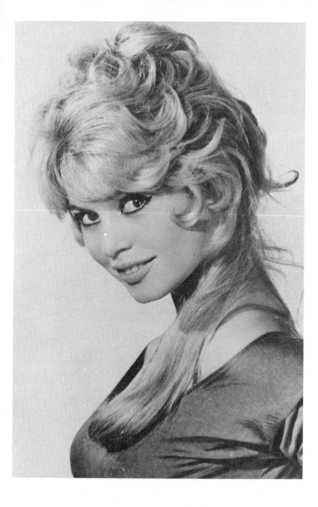
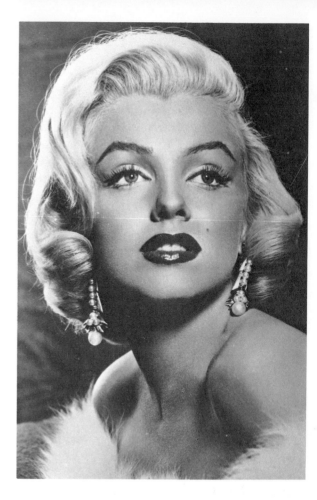
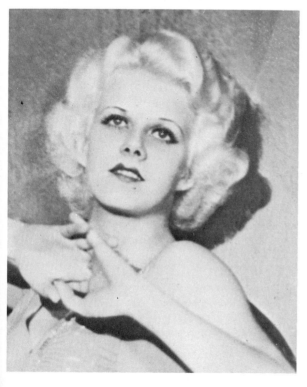
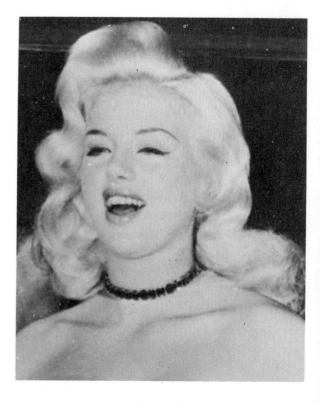

To understand this endocrine action and its relation to hair distribution in women, it is necessary to understand also the essential bisexuality or male-female potential of every creature born. There is a time between conception and birth when the primary organs of both sexes are present, and although the sex chromosomes sort this out and dictate the individual's sex before birth, the body never completely loses its bisexual potential. Every woman has potentially the same hair distribution as a man, the hair follicles for moustache, beard, and body hair all being present. Furthermore, her glands produce not only estrogen, the female hormone, but appreciable amounts of the male sex hormone, androgen. So long as the female balance is maintained, with estrogen dominant, everything, including hair growth and distribution, follows the normal female pattern. Occasionally, however, there is a balance that allows a slightly higher secretion of androgen, and if this occurs in a woman whose hair follicles are sensitive to even a very small amount of androgen, then hair growth is triggered and excess hair is produced. This condition is known as hirsutism. Both the glandular balance and the relative sensitivity are inherited factors and, as with male baldness, the only real answer to hirsutism is the sadly impracticable one of choosing one's parents.

Expert opinion now concedes that in the present state of our knowledge nothing can be done to prevent or cure hirsutism of this type. Estrogen administered as creams or as injections is no answer. Once the follicles have been triggered into action, no amount of estrogen will suppress them, and it may have unhappy side effects, including disturbance of the normal ovarian cycle. So for most women affected in this way the answer lies in shaving, which—contrary to popular belief—does not coarsen the growth; or in repeated bleaching, which can discourage it; or in electrolysis, which destroys the hair follicle.

Most women suffering from this problem are still completely feminine in every vital respect, and minor hirsutism is not really damaging to either appearance or confidence, if it is properly understood and dealt with. There is considerable comfort to be derived from some of the answers from men in our special survey. When asked how they reacted to surplus hair on women, one third said simply that they did not mind at all, saying something like "the girl is more important than the hair." One man admitted to feeling only jealousy. Another said that if, when a woman's clothes are removed, you find plenty of hair, "you have an energetic girl on your hands." (However, several of the more experienced males said they found hairy women no more sexy than others.) Some 5 per cent liked an excess of pubic hair, and one man expressed a definite preference

"For long periods the woman with blonde hair has been the object of the European male's desire."

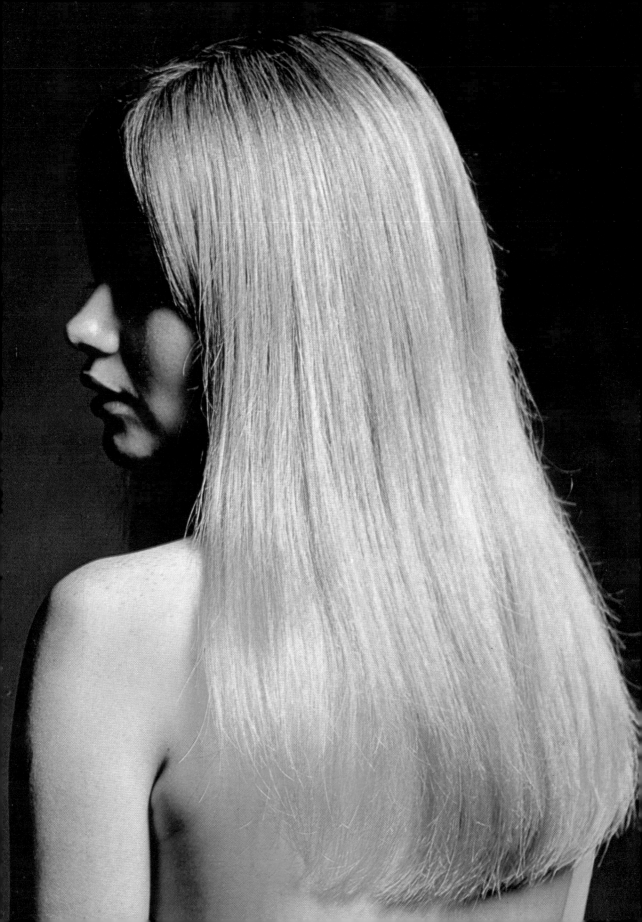

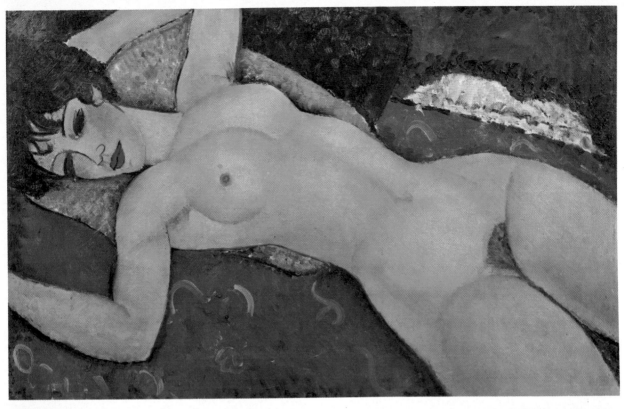

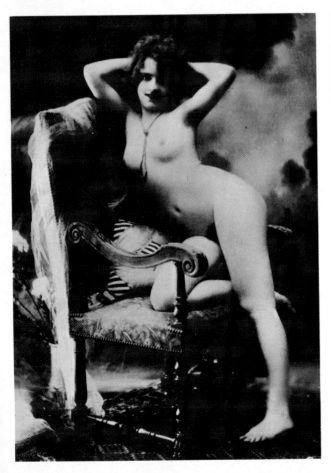

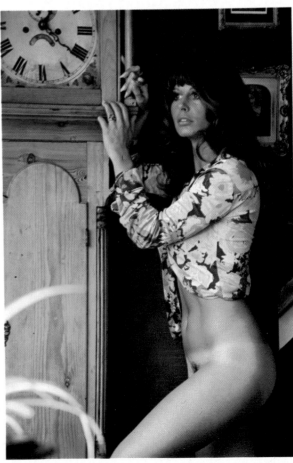

for hairy limbs. Two men were particularly attracted by facial hair, and several others had special tastes for hair on certain parts of a woman's body. All in all, it is clear that women with surplus hair are not at the sexual disadvantage they often assume.

The real tragedies are the rare cases of excessive hirsutism, including heavy growth on the arms, legs, breasts, and around the nipples, as well as a real moustache and beard. It is the more pitiful if the woman beneath all this is truly a woman, as is quite often the case. The bearded ladies of the side show and exhibition often have normal female curves, and bodies that produce babies. But hirsutism can sometimes be a by-product of a real masculinization of the body, resulting from congenital defects or the misfunction of the endocrine glands.

The tendency to grow a few facial hairs that some women develop at the menopause has the same underlying endocrine cause. With the onset of the menopause, the production of estrogen falls, allowing the balance to swing toward the androgens, which may trigger the growth of facial hair and occasionally cause the head hair to become sparser.

But for the vast majority of women whose hormonal balance is well within normal limits, endocrinology offers no answer to the subtle mystery of sexual potential, nor does the amount of hair a woman has on her head or body. The old myths and legends may be appealing, but the truth is that a woman's hair, or lack of hair, can affect her sex life only insofar as it affects her appearance or insofar as she *allows* it to affect her sexual response. If confidence is all-important to men, even more complex psychological factors determine women's sexual response. The most basic of these is the initial requirement of being found desirable.

But just what constitutes desirability so far as hair is concerned? It is particularly difficult to define this in relation to body hair, reactions to which vary far more widely than to head hair, both historically and geographically. Whereas head hair makes an almost universal appeal as at least potentially beautiful, body hair seems open to cultural preferences. This becomes less surprising if we consider other likes and dislikes. Arabs, for instance, account a double chin as one of their points in assessing beauty in a woman. Australian aborigines are fascinated by the charms of a very fat woman, however old and ugly she may be. In Polynesia, New Britain, and among some African tribes, young women, and in particular young brides, are especially fattened up. Eskimos and Kaffirs also much admire obesity, though the Kaffirs rationalize their preference by pointing out that a fat woman stands a better chance of weathering famine than a lean one. Hottentots and Bushmen go for enormous buttocks, now clearly

In depictions of the nude in art, pubic hair has often been discreetly concealed or omitted—with the result that when it is deliberately shown it may have an added shock erotic effect. Italian artist Amedeo Modigliani's Nude on a Cushion *(top), painted around 1917, owes some of its frank sexuality to its open display of pubic hair. In erotic art, pubic hair once had the attraction of the forbidden—as in the Edwardian photograph (bottom left) from* The Private Album of Count X. *The pin-up from modern men's magazine* Penthouse *(bottom right) still in 1970 permitted only a titillating glimpse of pubic hair.*

bred in by sexual selection, and many primitive tribes cut right across the more general taste for firm breasts by preferring pendant breasts so long that they permit a child carried on the back to be suckled.

Against this kind of background, widely differing attitudes to body hair seem perfectly understandable. Initially, as Man emerged as a thinking creature in a frightening and mysterious world, customs and attitudes were dictated by the mass of superstitions he built up to explain the inexplicable and to protect himself from the unseen powers ruling the natural elements and the lives of men. These attitudes and customs applied even to such comparative trivialities as hair and clothing, dictating which parts of the body should be covered, which uncovered. Later, of course, with growing sophistication and the long passage of the centuries, the original reasons were forgotten, but by then conditioning had fixed our responses and taught us, as it were, to like what we get. Obviously such built-in cultural preferences are open to modification, often under the dictates of a conquering race. (Sometimes, though, the conquered manage to impose upon the conqueror. Julius Caesar, for example, was more successful in forcing the Gauls to cut their hair than he was the obstinate Britons, and there is some evidence that Romans who settled in Britain eventually adopted the longer native hairstyle.)

In ancient Egypt neither men nor women allowed any body hair to remain; it was clearly thought to be both ugly and unhygienic. In ancient Greece complete depilation was the rule for women, always excepting head hair, although young boys, who presented the absolute ideal of beauty in a society where homosexuality without guilt was the order, were expected to remove hairs from their legs, but to retain their pubic hair, which was considered a thing of special delight. Mediterranean women, then as now, obviously had a strong growth of body hair, and to please their men were expected to remove it, or, perhaps, to shape at least their pubic hair by plucking, for the Athenian dramatist Aristophanes makes Lysistrata say:

> All we have to do is idly sit indoors
> With smooth roses powdered on our cheeks,
> Our bodies burning naked through the folds
> Of shining Imorgos' silk, and meet the men
> With our dear Venus plats plucked trim and neat:
> Their stirring love will rise up furiously,
> They'll beg our knees to open.

Greek influence had its effect on Rome, where it was a widespread custom to remove all hair from the body. No female statue of classical times shows pubic or axillary hair. One Roman emperor of the first

In spite of the appeal of the blonde, the vamp—the predatory and dangerous woman who challenges the male desire for sexual domination—is almost always dark-haired. The original screen vamp, Theda Bara (far right), made the most of the drama of black hair and black eyes. Modern sex symbol Raquel Welch (right) has a more natural look with a tumbling mass of brown hair.

century A.D., Domitian, whose public displays of cruelty were both subtle and excessive even for those terrible times, also had a strange taste in his more private moments and was reputed to spend long hours lying on a bed depilating his concubines' pubic regions with his own hand.

Women of the Turkish harems of much later times also had their pubic hair removed. An Italian traveler, Bassano de Zara, who visited Turkey in the mid-16th century, described how women of the harem decorated their bodies. "Some dye (with henna) the pubic region and four fingers' length above it. And for this reason they remove the hairs, considering it a sin to have any in the private parts."

Although Egyptian and Eastern customs may have influenced Greece, and Greece most surely influenced Rome, the same attitudes to body hair also arise quite spontaneously out of totally separate cultures, customs, and superstitions. The Dodingo of Uganda practiced depilation of all body hair, including the pubic. Special resins were applied and allowed to dry and then the whole pack, including hair, was simply torn away. It is a relief to learn that the skin was afterwards treated with soothing vegetable fats. Complete depilation of her body by the old women of the tribe was generally part of

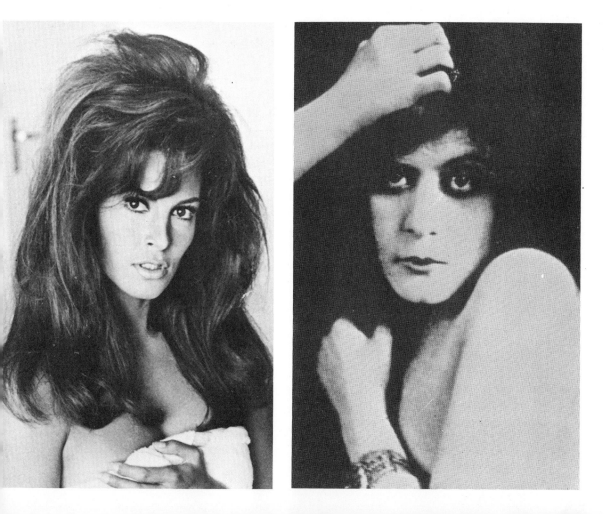

the preliminaries a young bride had to undergo before her wedding. The same custom existed in the Trobriand Islands, and was also widespread among South American Indians. Here there is an interesting suggestion that body hair was removed because the Indian considered brute creation so inferior to himself that he thought it degrading to resemble an animal in any way, even in hairiness.

Perhaps a similar kind of feeling explains why even sculptors from periods and places in which it was not the custom to remove body hair omitted it from their nudes of both men and women. Such artists as Michelangelo, Raphael, and Botticelli also omitted it in their paintings. Body hair was thought to emphasize the animal in us, and the idealized version of the human body either untruthfully omitted it or conveniently concealed it by a covering hand or drape. In the Middle Ages this may well have been dictated by the Church, which in the name of Christianity invested sex with an aura of guilt for almost 2000 years. But some artists feel that if a nude woman is painted with her pubic hair as it exists in nature, all eyes are drawn to this region instead of taking in the beauty of the whole body.

There is no record of pubic hair at any time being considered sexually unattractive by Europeans. The normal European attitude is summed up in this passage—actually written by Alexander Trocchi—from Frank Harris's *My Life and Loves,* describing a Eurasian girl who had been procured for Harris. "Her lips were smooth and rounded and gave downwards to a pair of soft and shapely thighs on which the hairless mound, naked of hair between their roundnesses, jutted outwards like a soft beak. I must say I found that rather ugly. It is a fallacy to think that a woman's sexual organ is less prominent when it is shaven of its hair. The hair, rising as it does outwards and away from the lower belly, has a tendency to obscure the sharpness of the line of the mound, thus rendering the mount itself less prominent, more subtle in its provocativeness and more modest to a man's lips. Hair is the grass of the human body, the verdure and the beauty of the carnal meadow."

The "grass" metaphor is, of course, not new. Shakespeare uses it in *Venus and Adonis* in two verses that make the charms of a woman's body hair to the Elizabethans subtly but delightfully clear:

> "Fondling" she saith, "since I have hemm'd thee here,
> Within the circuit of this ivory pale
> I'll be a park, and thou shalt be my deer;
> Feed where thou wilt, on fountain or in dale;
> Graze on my lips; and if those hills be dry
> Stray lower, where the pleasant fountains lie.

The number of things a woman can do with her pubic hair to improve on nature is strictly limited. She may draw attention to it by semi-concealing it—as Lucas Cranach half-hid the hair of his Eve *(top left)—under "see-through" panties (top right). She may cover it completely by wearing a G-string (center right). She may shave it, or trim it to a different shape—such as the heart shape once advocated by Mary Quant (bottom left). Or she may artificially add to it by wearing a pubic wig—in this case (bottom right) of fur.*

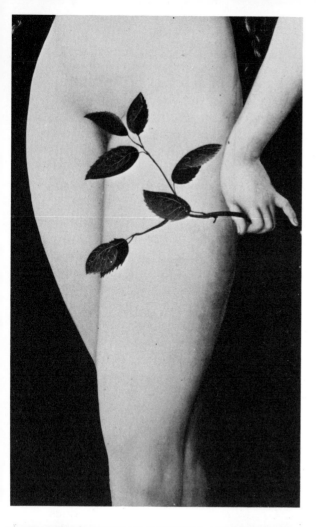

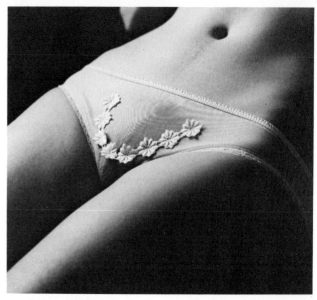

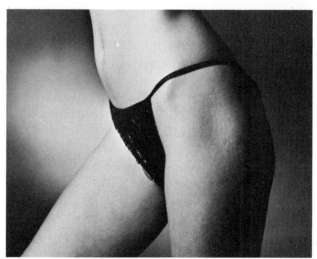

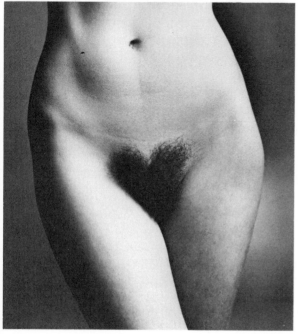

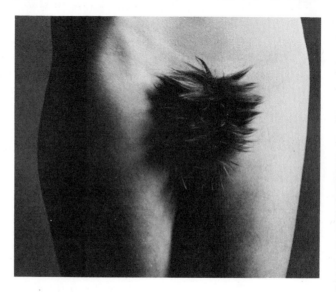

"Within this limit is relief enough,
Sweet bottom-grass, and high delightful plain,
Round rising hillocks, brakes obscure and rough,
To shelter thee from tempest and from rain;
Then be my deer, since I am such a park;
No dog shall rouse thee, tho' a thousand bark."

Assessing contemporary attitudes to women's body hair in a real sexual context is not easy. Our special survey again throws a little light on how some sexually experienced men feel about it. Out of the total male sample, about 25 per cent were excited by the sight of a woman's axillary hair (in one case "if an older woman, because it's slightly obscene"). Two men found it more exciting than pubic hair. Nearly three quarters of the men preferred that their girl friends should remove axillary hair; only 16 per cent came down on the opposite side and preferred it not to be shaved. All the women except three did in fact regularly shave off their axillary hair, and those three refrained to please their partners. Sixty-five per cent of the men were aroused—some to erection—by the sight of female pubic hair. Only four of them wanted their partners to remove their pubic hair, one on grounds of hygiene, another simply because he had pictured women as hairless and had been shocked when he first saw a naked girl.

Men's reaction to women's pubic hair seems to depend, in fact, not so much on its aesthetic or sexual attractions as on their own inhibitions. The extremes can be illustrated by two examples, one real and one fictional. John Ruskin, the 19th-century English critic and reformer, was so shocked by the sight of his wife's pubic hair on their wedding night that he became impotent. Just before the marriage was annulled, in 1854, Mrs. Ruskin wrote to her father, relating the sad story of her marriage. Ruskin had refused to consummate the marriage "and finally this last year told me his true reason (and this to me is as villainous as all the rest) that he had imagined women were quite different to what he saw I was, and the reason he did not make me his wife was because he was disgusted with my person the first evening . . . ." It is difficult to imagine anything more remote from this than the behavior of Mellors, the gamekeeper of D. H. Lawrence's novel *Lady Chatterley's Lover:*

". . . he looked at the folds of her body in the fire-glow, and at the fleece of soft brown hair that hung down to a point between her open thighs. He reached to the table behind, and took up her bunch of flowers, still so wet that drops of rain fell on to her . . . .

With quiet fingers he threaded a few forget-me-not flowers in the fine brown fleece of the mound of Venus.

'There!' he said. 'There's forget-me-nots in the right place!'

She looked down at the milky odd little flowers among the brown maiden-hair at the lower tip of her body.

'Doesn't it look pretty!' she said.

'Pretty as life,' he replied.

And he stuck a pink campion-bud among the hair.

'There! That's me where you won't forget me! That's Moses in the bullrushes'."

Women themselves seem convinced that their pubic hair is a powerful weapon in their sexual armory—or so thought 80 per cent of the women questioned in our survey. Three of them found it to be a stimulant so strong that it led to instant erection in the male. Only $12\frac{1}{2}$ per cent found their pubic hair unexciting to the male. The very few women who shaved or shaped it did so at the request of their partners.

So, in the intimate matter of body hair, women seem to try to please men. With head hair, the story has been very different. Here the desires of men have come a poor second to the demands of fashion. And, similarly, men in their turn have only rarely been influenced by women in their choice of style for head and facial hair.

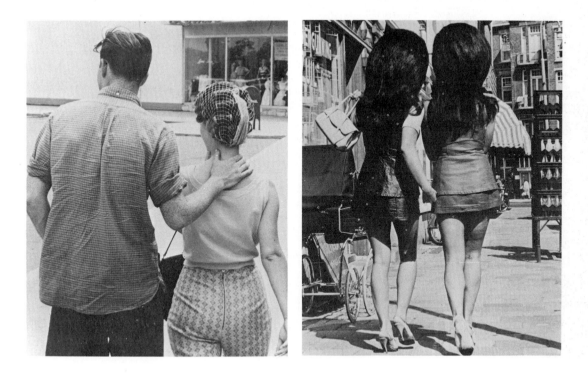

Men have always preferred women's hair to be loose and natural-looking, but women have consistently ignored men's wishes and yielded instead to the demands of fashion. Left, a woman in curlers walks with her escort in a US shopping precinct. Right, top-heavy bouffant hair styles disproportionately exaggerated by miniskirts.

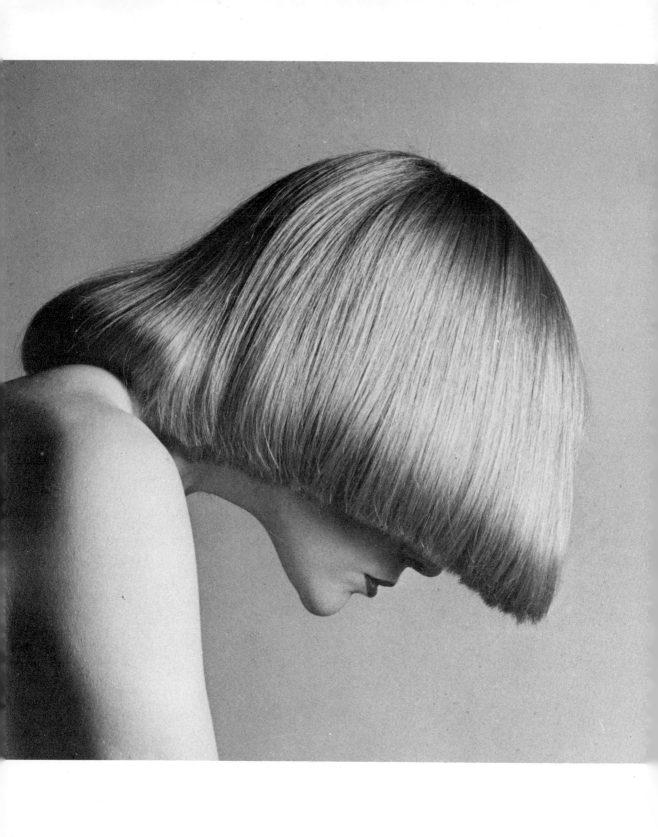

4 *Fashion and Display*

Once the human race discovered that hair was good-tempered, pliable, and regenerative, and could be cut, shaved, shaped, dyed, braided, crimped, curled, waved, puffed, padded, and frizzed, it proceeded to use hair in a vast variety of permutations of length, style, and color, in the long, continuous search for novelty, beauty, and status sometimes called fashion.

If the search had been concerned only with beauty, it would all have been much simpler. Then it would have been just a matter of individual choice, of fitting a hair style to a face to emphasize the good points, disguise the bad, and make a more harmonious whole. When, on rare occasions, hair has been used in this way, it has been a face-saver for the plain woman and a head-turner for the beautiful.

But much more often beauty has been only a secondary consideration and hair styles, for both men and women, have been ways of proclaiming status through novelty. A style was introduced by an accepted leader of fashion, often a king or his mistress, and—however hideous—was admired and followed, partly to flatter its author, and partly to proclaim membership in an elite circle. For fashion, whether in hair, clothes, or manners, has only ever really concerned the elite—the privileged members of court and society, and a few wealthy hangers-on. As the middle classes emerged, it is true, fashions sometimes lasted long enough to percolate down and be copied by them, but a successful fashion carries within it the seed of its own destruction. For as soon as it is no longer a novelty, as soon as it becomes commonplace, it is time for it to be superseded. How otherwise can the elite be distinguished?

Things are changing, of course. Once, hair styles were deliberately kept so complex and ornate that only the wealthy with much time on their

Expensive simplicity—a hair style of the late 1960s.

hands could afford to display them. It is significant that loose, natural-looking hair has hardly ever been worn by fashionable women, although men have always thought it infinitely more desirable and attractive than a complicated, formal hair style. Its adoption would have denied these women an absorbing pastime for their empty lives, and would also have approximated too closely to styles worn by the common people.

Today, with sharp social distinctions fading, and with a wide range of hairdressers at a wide range of prices replacing ladies' maids and exclusive hair stylists, most women in the developed countries can share the thrills and hazards of fashionable hair. Home permanent waves and inexpensive, safe color rinses have opened wide the gates to experiment, and the mass media can flash the fashion message around the world to ensure the most rapid turnover ever in styles.

It is not royalty today that is the leader in hair fashion, although America's "royalty," Jacqueline Kennedy, certainly set a trend: her hair

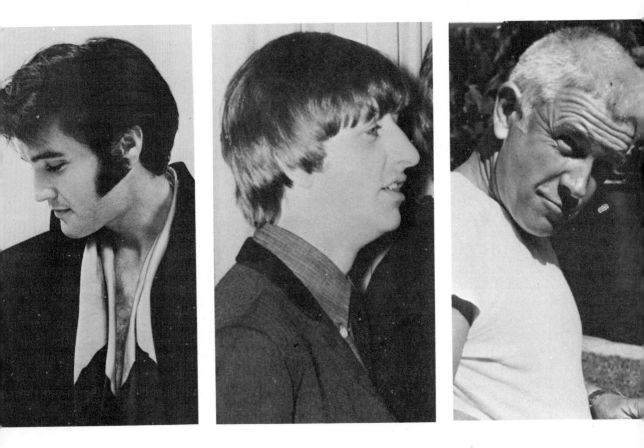

In the late 1950s and 1960s longer hair styles—like those of US singer and movie star Elvis Presley (left) and British Beatle Ringo Starr (center)—began to challenge the short crewcut that had for many years been the accepted norm for men.

style was copied in thousands of small salons on unlikely faces. Hair fashions now are devised by the top hairdressers and displayed by mass media's own royalty, the actresses, film stars, and pop singers. Veronica Lake, the Hollywood star of the forties, doomed her followers to grope about behind a curtain of hair in a one-eyed world. Brigitte Bardot popularized the tousled look. The film stars Audrey Hepburn and Mia Farrow promoted gamine and urchin cuts, while four young Liverpudlians from England had a runaway success, not just with their music, but with the Beatle haircut. If that seemed wild and eccentric in the early sixties, it was to seem positively conservative compared with the frantic, unkempt locks of pop groups such as the Rolling Stones and the Kinks, or the fuzzed-out style of a pop musician such as the late Jimi Hendrix.

These modern setters of hair fashion are usually concerned with establishing an image, something that will have impact on their audiences. In the past, fashions were devised and followed for different reasons. In the second century A.D., the emperor Hadrian grew a beard to conceal some scars. Because he was emperor, other Romans copied him, and so the fashion of wearing beards was reintroduced after some 400 years of mostly beardless men. When, in 1461, illness forced Duke Philip of Burgundy to have his hair shaved off, 500 noblemen followed suit. In 1521, a minor accident to one man sent a good part of the Western world to its barbers. One winter evening, Francis I, king of France, with several of his favorites, stormed the house of Count Montgomery with snowballs. A flaming torch, flung to ward off the playful invasion, wounded the king on the head. To treat the injury, the king's doctors cut his hair short. His courtiers tactfully adopted the same shorter style, and so the rush to the barbers began. Henry VIII of England, impressed by the new French style, decided to wear it himself, and in 1535 commanded his courtiers to follow suit.

Beards, moustaches, and whiskers have been in and out of fashion like the tide throughout history, although rather less predictably. The cult of the elite was at work here too—very evidently in ancient Greece and Rome, where if the fashion was for beards, then slaves must be clean-shaven, and if it was fashionable to be clean-shaven, then the slaves must grow beards. Facial hair had its leaders, and its eccentrics. Alexander the Great is credited with setting a fashion for clean-shaven chins that was to last in Greece for almost 1000 years. The ancient Greeks had usually worn beards, but in 323 B.C., Alexander ordered his armies to shave so that the Persians could not use his soldiers' beards as handles in battle.

Not just any beard, but special styles of beard and whiskers were made popular by different men at different times. The Emperor Napoleon III of France adopted a small beard, known as an "imperial," which was widely admired and copied; the Union general Benjamin Franklin Kelley introduced the "Uncle Sam" beard in the United States; and the last German Kaiser gave his name to a particular, rather solid-looking moustache. At least one sort of whiskers, "Dundrearies," took their name from a fictional character, Lord Dundreary, in *Our American Cousin*—the play President Lincoln was attending when he was assassinated in 1865. "Burnsides" (sometimes reversed to "sideburns"), a heavy growth of side-whiskers curving across the cheek to join the moustache, took their name from whiskers worn by another Union general, Ambrose Burnside, in the American Civil War.

There has been almost as much variety in beards and whiskers as in hair styles, and no doubt it has all added up to good trade for the barbers. Beard styles listed by an English Puritan, Philip Stubbes, in *The Anatomie of Abuses* (1583) included: the French, Spanish, Dutch, Italian, new, old, bravado, mean, gentlemen's, common, court, and country. But others evolved with more imaginative names. The "cathedral," worn by John Knox, the Scottish religious reformer, in the 16th century, took its name from its popularity with churchmen. Other names were more directly descriptive. The "sugar-loaf" was long and rounded, but wider at the top than at the bottom. Names such as "forked," "spade," "swallow-tail," "bush," "stiletto," "needle," "Roman T," "screw," and "fantail" all indicated shape. Beards were dyed, curled, waved, crisped, frizzed, plaited, matted, braided, and even crisscrossed. They were oiled, perfumed, waxed, powdered, and sprinkled with gold dust. They were loved and loathed, honored and reviled, commanded, forbidden, and even taxed.

The leaders of women's hair fashions were frequently the great courtesans of the day. The Duchesse de Fontanges, a mistress of Louis XIV of France, gave her name to a hair style created by accident in about 1680. Out hunting with Louis one day, the duchess lost her hat and tied up her curls with a lace-edged garter. The king declared the effect delightful, and a new mode was launched. The "fontange," as it was called, soon developed into a high tower of lace and ribbons stretched on wire, which at its most exaggerated brushed chandeliers and caused doorways to be heightened and the roofs of carrying chairs to be raised all over Europe. (Perhaps fortunately, the charming Lady Sandwich, wife of the English ambassador, was presented at the French court in 1714 wearing a simple and becoming low coiffure. This ended the popularity of the "fontange," and also, so it is said, the prosperity of the lace-makers.) Madame de Pompadour, a mistress of Louis XV, gave her name to a particular fashion still called after her, but

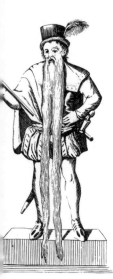

Hans Steiniger, a burgomaster of Braunau, Austria, whose beard was longer than he was. The fame it brought him was dearly earned: in 1567 he tripped over it while going up to the council chamber, tumbled down the stairs, and was killed.

it was written of her: "A hundred entrancing ways did she arrange her hair—now powdered, now in all its own silken glory, now brushed straight back, ears showing, now in curls on her neck—till the court nearly went mad attempting to imitate her inimitable coiffures."

Marie Antoinette, the wife of Louis XVI, may be said to have made the most of her head while she had it. Going to a ball in 1776, according to the 19th-century American periodical, *Godey's Lady's Book,* she "had a headdress so high she could not get into her carriage, and it was therefore taken off, and replaced when she arrived. All headdresses, however, could not be taken to pieces in this way, and the ladies, victims of vanity, were forced to keep their heads out of the window of their carriages, and sometimes even to kneel." After the birth of her last child, Marie Antoinette's fair hair began to fall out; then, because of an illness, she had to have it cut short. All the court copied her new simple style, "à l'enfant." Yet the queen preferred, when she could, to have her own hair elaborately built up, using false hair for padding. Her favorite style, "à la Minerve," required no less than 10 ostrich feathers.

But Marie Antoinette was restrained compared with some of her contemporaries. No period produced such preposterous and grotesque extravaganzas of hair as the 18th century. A certain Madame de Lauzun reached perhaps the most absurd extreme by wearing an enormously high headdress of hair and artificial hair, on top of which were modeled ducks swimming in a stormy sea, scenes of hunting and shooting, a mill with a miller's wife flirting with a priest, and the miller leading an ass by its halter. Skilled coiffeurs were needed to erect the more and more outrageous styles, and once up, they were not disturbed for many weeks. As the interior was filled with wool, tow, and hemp, plastered together with a "pomatum" based on beef marrow, the smell gradually became anything but alluring. Needless to say, men protested, and one form was a newspaper ode printed in 1768:

> When he scents the mingled steam
> Which your plaster'd heads are rich in,
> Lard and meal, and clouted cream,
> Can he love a walking kitchen?

Even worse than the smell, perhaps, was the animal life the "walking kitchens" harbored. A letter published in 1768 in the *London Magazine* protested against "the present prodigious, unnatural, monstrous, and dirty mode of dressing the hair," and went on to describe what the writer had seen when his elderly aunt's head had been "opened up." Swarms of "animalculas" were running around, but the coiffeur assured him they

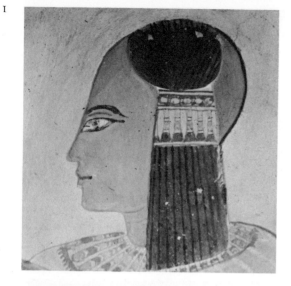

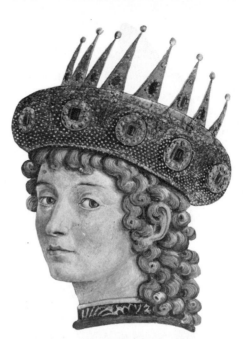

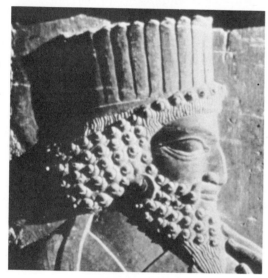

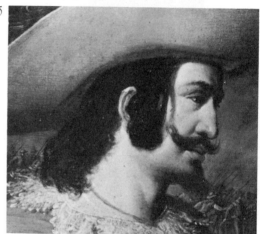

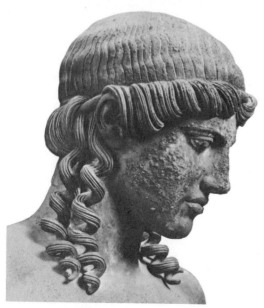

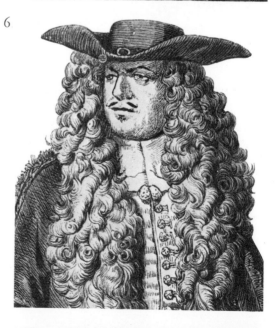

7

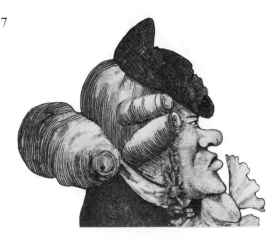

10

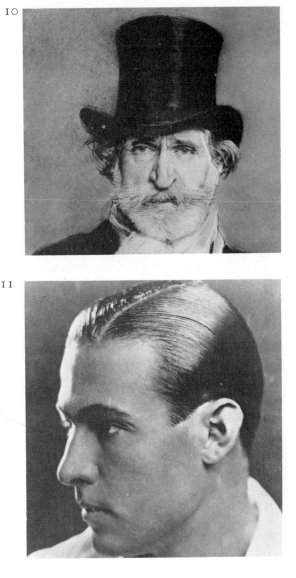

8

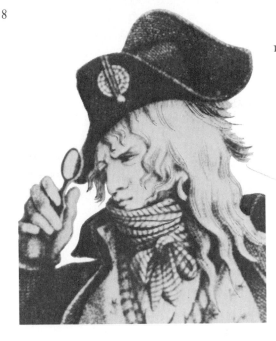

11

9

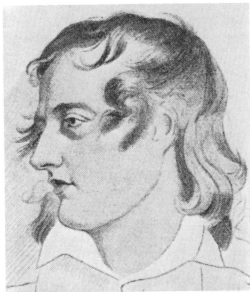

Men's hair styles through the ages. *1.* tomb painting of the young son of Rameses III of Egypt (12th century B.C.) *2.* a Persian officer in the army of Darius the Great (521–486 B.C.). *3.* a bronze head of Apollo from the 5th-century B.C.—a typical hair style of a Greek youth of the time. *4.* Lorenzo the Magnificent wearing his hair in a court style of 15th-century Florence. *5.* a Spanish gentleman of about 1640, when Spain led European fashion. *6.* bust by Gian Lorenzo Bernini of Francis I d'Este wearing a luxuriant mid-17th-century wig. *7.* a Macaroni of the late 18th-century. *8.* caricature of a young French dandy of about 1796. *9.* the Romantic image of the early 19th century exemplified by Lord Byron. *10.* the bearded but disciplined later 19th-century look shown by Italian composer Giuseppe Verdi. *11.* Rudolph Valentino, US sex-symbol of the 1920s, who popularized the patent-leather look.

could not migrate to other parts of the body as they were held fast in the glutinous matter formed by the pomatum. Other reports have described nests of mice being discovered, and clearly the elegant ivory "scratchers" of the period, mounted on long sticks, were of more than ornamental value. Men really had something to protest about. But then, they had always protested, even when they had far less cause. In *The Anatomie of Abuses,* Philip Stubbes had attacked Elizabethan women's fashions on moral rather than hygienic grounds:

"If curling and laying out their owne naturall haire were all (which is impious, and at no hande lawfull, being, as it is, an ensigne of pride, and the standerd of wantonnesse to all that behold it), it were the lesse matter; but thei are not simplie content with their owne haire, but buye other haire, either of horses, mares, or any other straunge beastes, dying it of what colour they list themselves. . . . So whereas their haire was given them as a signe of subjection, and therefore they were commaunded to cherish the same, now have they made it an ornament of pride, and destruction to themselves for ever, excepte they repent."

But women have at no time been repentant. Much the same complaint was made in the third century by the Christian ecclesiastical writer Tertullian: "All this wasted pain on arranging your hair—what contribution can this make to your salvation? Why can you not give your hair a rest? One minute you are building it up, the next you are letting it down—raising it one moment, stretching it the next . . . ."

Tertullian was not the only one to complain about Roman fashions. Martial, 200 years earlier, had written an epigram about Messalina, the notoriously unfaithful wife of the Emperor Claudius: "Her toilet table contained a hundred lies; and while she was in Rome, her hair was blushing by the Rhine." This was a reference to the habit of wearing wigs and false hair, particularly fair hair purchased from Gaul. In a gibe at another woman, Martial wrote:

The golden hair that Galla wears
Is hers—who would have thought it?
She swears 'tis hers, and true she swears,
For I know where she bought it.

And Ovid, writing at about the time of Christ, in his *Art of Love,* made fun of a lady who was in such a fluster at his unexpected arrival that she put on her wig back-to-front.

Despite the protests men have made against the worst excesses and mutilations that fashions have dictated for women's hair, they have not been immune themselves. In ancient Rome, men lavished ointments and oil on

Women's hair styles through the ages. 1. an Etruscan woman of the court. 2. head of a Roman lady of the late 1st century A.D. 3. the late-medieval plucked look in a painting by Roger van der Weyden (1400–64). 4. portrait by Piero di Cosimo of Simonetta Vespucci—a lady of the Italian Renaissance. 5. La Bella Ferronière, by Leonardo da Vinci (about 1517). 6. an English lady of the early 18th century, painted by Thomas Gainsborough.

1

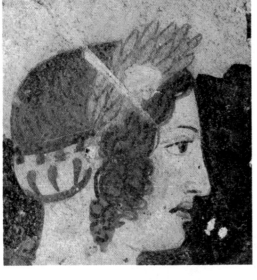

2

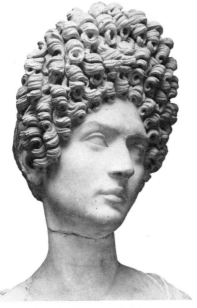

3

4

5

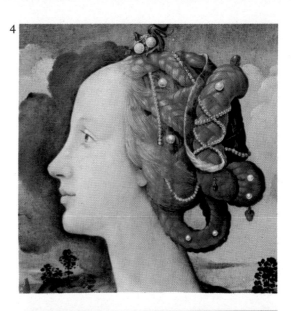

6

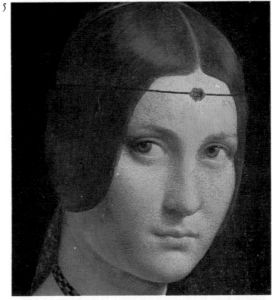

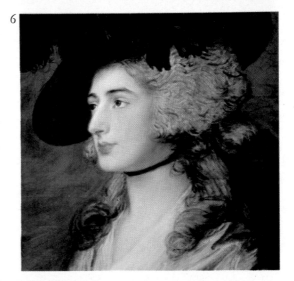

7

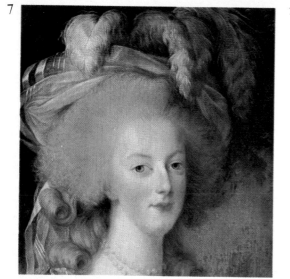

10

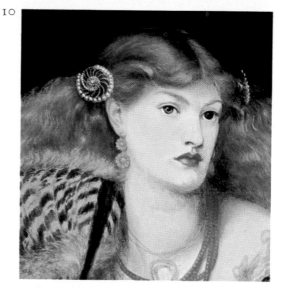

8

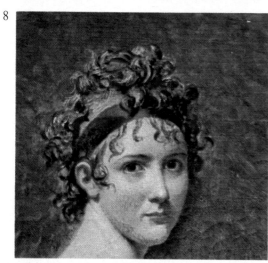

11

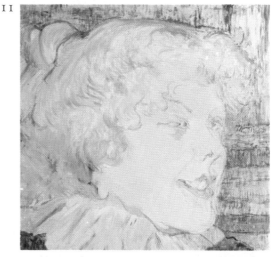

9

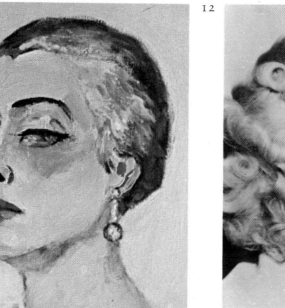

12

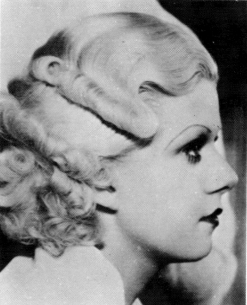

both head and beard and, according to Cicero in the first century B.C., were not above tinting their hair as well. In the luxurious days of the later Roman Empire, gold dust was used by several of the emperors, including Commodus in the second century A.D., whose hair was described by the historian Herodian as glittering "from its natural whiteness and from the quantity of essences and gold dust with which it was loaded."

Meanwhile, the peoples whom the Romans regarded as barbarians were not without pride in their hair. The Gauls bleached their hair with a solution containing chalk. Anglo-Saxon men dyed their hair and beards blue, or sometimes green or orange, thus setting a sporadic fashion for hair shades outside the natural range. At varying times, pink, blue, and violet powders later became popular in Europe. Finally, at the beginning of the 18th century, white became the smart powder for young men as well as old. It was applied both to natural hair, often built up to heights that rivaled those of the ladies, and to the enormous wigs that by this time had become popular.

The full-bottomed wig, which reached almost to the waist, was as grotesque as anything the ladies dreamed up. In 1717, in Sir John Vanbrugh's comedy *The Relapse,* a wig-maker assures Lord Foppington that his new wig is "so long and full of hair, it may serve you for a Hat and Cloak in all weathers," and Lord Foppington comments that "a Perriwig to a man shou'd be like a Mask to a Woman: nothing shou'd be seen but his Eyes." Men carried combs and mirrors, and combed their wigs quite publicly. Like women they sought novelty in absurdity, and around 1770 a group of young men who had spent some time in Italy introduced what came to be called the Macaroni style, an exaggeratedly high toupee built up on wire frames or cushions of wool or felt.

Of course, the vanity and worldliness of hair fashions was always being challenged. Both Church and State at different times in history tried to influence styles through edicts, legislation, taxes, threats, and pulpit thunderings. Clemens Romanus, the first of the Apostolic Fathers, urged men "to pole their Heads, and not to suffer their Haire to grow long, lest the nourishing and perfuming of their Haire should be a meanes to inflame their lusts, and to illaqueate or inamour women with them"— which sounds the argument least likely to succeed.

The early Christian Church disapproved of wigs, and the wearing of them was declared by some churchmen to be a mortal sin. Tertullian, who was a fanatic, declared that "all personal disguise is adultery before God. All perukes, paint, and powder are such disguises and inventions of the devil . . . ." Moreover, he warned, "the fake hair you wear may have

7. Marie Antoinette in 1784. 8. Madame Recamier, a leader of fashion in early 19th-century France. 9. a short mannish style of the 1920s. 10. the Pre-Raphaelites set a vogue for long, supposedly "medieval" hair styles like that in this portrait by Dante Gabriel Rossetti (1828–1882). 11. L'Anglaise du Star by Henri Toulouse-Lautrec (1864–1901)—a style of the late 19th century. 12. the groomed, permanently waved look of Hollywood in the 1930s.

come not only from a criminal but from a very dirty head, perhaps from the head of one already damned." The theologian Clement of Alexandria clinched the argument by pronouncing that when anyone wearing a wig was blessed, the benediction remained on the wig, and did not penetrate to the wearer.

Inside the Church the struggle to regulate the length of hair and beards went on. In the seventh century a fierce difference of opinion between the Catholic Church of England, Scotland, and Ireland, and the See of Rome, ended with victory for the pope, who insisted that the use of the razor was indispensable to salvation. Thereafter, priests not only shaved all but a ring of hair from their heads, but wore neither beard nor whiskers. By the ninth century, all was confusion again, with Catholic priests wearing beards (and some not even shaving the head), while the Greek Church remained clean-shaven. A few centuries later, Catholic priests were again forced to shave, while the Greeks became happily bearded, and still remain so. From Clement VII (1523), even the popes went bearded, until Clement XI in 1700, who began the present shaven series.

The Church's confusion affected laymen as well as priests. Any long-haired penitent kneeling before the 11th-century Bishop of Worcester, St. Wulfstan, received more than a blessing; he got a free haircut too, with the bishop wielding the knife. In 1096 the Archbishop of Rouen proclaimed that anyone wearing long hair or a beard should be excluded from the Church, both before and after death. In 1102 a decree in Venice banned long beards, and on Christmas Day in 1105 the Bishop of Amiens refused communion to anyone wearing a beard. In the same year, Bishop Serlo of Seez in Normandy not only convinced Henry I of England, in a hell-fire sermon, of the evil of long hair and beards, but promptly produced a pair of scissors from his vestments and sheared the king there and then. Needless to say, Henry's courtiers followed the fashion.

Beards have at various times suffered secular as well as religious attack. In England during the brief reign of Edward VI (1547–53), commoners were prohibited from wearing a beard of more than three weeks' growth, under penalty of a 40-shilling fine. In 1558, in the first year of Elizabeth's reign, a tax was imposed on beards according to the age and social standing of the owner. It proved unpopular and unenforceable, and was repealed in the following year, ushering in the arrogant beards of the Elizabethan age. Perhaps the most determined taxing of beards was in Russia, where Peter the Great, as part of his campaign to westernize Russia (and to obtain useful revenue), imposed in 1698 a tax of 100 roubles on bearded noblemen, with a sliding scale for lower ranks. Tax collectors waylaid travelers at the gates of towns, issuing beard licenses in the form of copper disks. If the traveler could not or would not pay, his beard was often forcibly removed.

One hair tax that had wide political repercussions was imposed in England in 1795. It was a tax on hair powder, introduced to raise funds for the war against Napoleon. It brought in comparatively little revenue. Many men gave up powdering their hair rather than pay, for it was a period in which disastrous harvests caused hungry mobs to raise a bitter outcry against the waste of flour for hair powder. Not for the first time, hair became a political issue. The Tories, who had sponsored the tax, demonstrated their principles by paying up and continuing to wear powder on their heads and wigs. Some of them, as a gesture of defiance, powdered their dogs and horses also. Whigs began to wear short hair—unpowdered.

Earlier, in the 17th century, the same sort of thing had happened during the English Revolution. The Puritan followers of Cromwell wore their hair cropped short, and were known as Roundheads, while the Cavaliers, or Royalists, continued to wear their hair very long, using wigs if necessary to achieve the defiant effect. Again, moral indignation and moral sanctions were the main weapons against long hair, and Pastor Thomas Hall of Kingsnorton wrote in 1653 a long screed on *The Loathsomnesse of Long Haire*.

Even the New World took up the battle. In 1649, Governor Dudley of the Bay Colony issued an alarmed proclamation against the invasion of long hair "after the manner of ruffians and barbarous Indians." He and the magistrates signing it declared their "dislike and detestation against the wearing of such long hair, as against a thing uncivil and unmanly . . . ." It was in America, too, that future Congregationalist clergyman and leader Cotton Mather in 1683 castigated women as "apes of Fancy, frizaling and curlying of their hayr," and urged them to refrain from pride in false locks and "towers like comets about their heads." Nathaniel Ward, who drew up New England's first code of laws, showed a certain flair for picturesque imagery by rebuking styles like "ill-shapen, shotten shell-fish, Egyptian hieroglyphics, or at the best . . . French flurts of the pastry."

So much feeling and so much indignation over the centuries about little bits of hair on the face or the length of hair on the head! It is impossible not to feel that all that energy might have been better employed fighting the very real injustices and abuses of the times. Attempts to regulate appearance seem the more strange to us in a period when the concept of personal freedom and the cult of the individual are part of at least the democratic societies. And yet we cannot be too complacent, for we are now seeing the older section of society protesting strongly against the reintroduction by young men of the fashion for long hair.

This chapter has not given space to all the many different and fascinating styles and variations in hair, beards, and moustaches over the centuries. For those interested, this has already been done by Richard Corson in his scholarly book *Fashions in Hair* (1965), which must surely stand as the definitive work for a long time to come. What has not been done, and is interesting to attempt, is to relate the broad trends and major changes in hair styles at certain key periods in history to changing social conditions and sexual mores. Hair on occasions has been a banner that has both asserted and reflected truths about society.

Although we have seen how the pressures of Church and State have influenced hair styles, and how individual leaders have set the fashion, it is still fascinating to speculate why, at certain points in time, people have adopted new fashions, reacting against the current trend instead of conforming to it. Neither manners, morals, nor hair styles evolve in a vacuum.

If only because most of us have been eyewitnesses, it is simplest first to consider recent styles, and especially the current vogue for long hair among young men, and loose, straight, natural-looking hair among girls. In both cases, there is a clear reaction against existing predominant styles—against male crew-cut conformity, and against female permanent waves, curls, and bogus Hollywood glamor. This is the scene the young reject, and they display this rejection in their hair styles.

The sexual connotations of the issue of short versus long hair are strong. In *The Unconscious Significance of Hair,* Charles Berg made a great point of linking haircutting with castration and denial of sexual freedom, and long hair with the acceptance and enjoyment of sexuality. The long, loose hair of girls today, and the almost blatant hairiness of young men, would appear to confirm his theory, for this generation has a frank appreciation of sex. Removal of religious sanctions, a more profound understanding of our sexual natures, and above all, for the first time in history, a fully effective method of contraception have all led to a change in sexual mores clearly reflected in hair fashions.

There is another interesting phenomenon in modern society that current hair styles tend to reflect. This is the blurred role of the sexes. Education and emancipation have given women improved status and financial independence. The Pill has given them sexual independence. For the first time, they can approach sexual experience, if they wish, as men have always been free to do, as something divorced from procreation. The old double standards and hypocrisies have been swept away, so that young men and women have something approaching real equality. Both are wage earners, even after marriage. Both expect sexual fulfillment, and if they do not find it within marriage, reserve the right to look for it outside. Future generations looking back at the hair styles of the late sixties and seventies must see this blurring of roles reflected in the hair, often almost indistinguishable between the sexes, of young men and women. It is not without cause that this has become in clothes and hair the age of unisex.

Another indication of the changing social pattern of this age, which can be read in the latest hair gimmick, is the emergence in the USA of an independent, proud, and militant black culture. The idealistic young have flocked to support the Civil Rights movement, and young whites proudly wear the new Afro hair style, asserting their belief in the essential equality of man, as well as hinting at sexual power, through the style's suggestion of Negro virility and its resemblance in type to coarse, curly pubic hair. The young have let their hair down with a vengeance and a purpose, and they are reveling in it. In no previous age could a musical called *Hair*, with a young cast beating out a wild erotic message, have so surely caught on with the public from New York to London, and from Tokyo to Los Angeles. The central song, with the dancers shaking and twirling their magnificent manes, is a positive hymn to hair:

> There ain't no words for the beauty,
>   the splendor, the wonder of my
> Hair, hair, hair, hair, hair, hair, hair, hair,
> Flow it, show it, long as God can grow it, my hair.
> I want it long, straight, curly, fuzzy, snaggy, shaggy,
> Ratty, matty, oily, greasy, fleecy, shining,
>   gleaming, steaming,
> Flaxen, waxen, knotted, polka dotted,
> Twisted, beaded, braided, powdered, flowered
>   and confettied,
> Bangled, tangled, spangled and spaghettied.

It will be interesting to see if, once again, there is a move back to restraint. If so, and if it is to succeed and tilt the seesaw of fashion once again, then it may well come from among the young themselves, not be imposed from outside. There have already been some signs of this in the eruption of the skinhead movement in Britain, but this will be discussed in the next chapter. What will almost certainly survive and grow is the need for men to adopt the "peacock" role. Now that women are so much more independent, and the sex ratio of births is in their favor, men must once more set out to attract. Women can pick and choose, and where there is choice there must be variety. Long hair is the passport to variety, and so the chances are that it will continue and eventually gain acceptance.

Prediction is obviously difficult and dangerous and the swing-back could come at any time. A new pop star could start it, or it could rise out of a sudden revulsion against anarchistic tendencies within society. It is safer, perhaps, to look back and see how social movements have been reflected in the hair fashions of other periods. One period when female fashions were a banner for all to see was the 1920s. Hobble skirts, long hair, buns, and hat pins had been blown out of existence by World War I. Women had proved they could do jobs and take responsibility, and they were to be rewarded with the vote. At last, it seemed, they were to be the equal of men, and it went straight to their heads. In mistaken enthusiasm they tried to look like men, even to the point of the Eton crop. It takes little imagination to realize that those short dresses, cropped heads, and flat chests were the immediate reaction to emancipation.

In Victorian England, ladies' hair, with its braids, ribbons, plaits, and puffs, was as constrained as their lives, with nothing loose or free. But in the heavy beards and side-whiskers of the men there seemed to be a strong assertion of the male authority and parental power that characterized the age. And it is possible, also, to wonder if thrusting beards and pronounced facial hair might be an expression of a confident and dynamic period. England in the 19th century was reaping the rich rewards of the Industrial Revolution at home, and of the Empire overseas. She was confident in benign Providence, a just God, Queen Victoria, the upper classes, paternalism, and the superiority of a white skin, particularly if it was British. Enemies might rattle their sabers across the Channel or in South Africa, but they would not prevail. The same kind of dynamic society and confidence existed in Elizabethan England, when there was also a great display of beards and moustaches. The styles may have been different, but it is possible that the unconscious motivation was the same.

Conversely, the stupid, impractical, elaborate hair structures of the 18th century tell their own story of vain and empty lives, of self-indulgence and boredom, which had to be relieved by the constant pursuit of novelty. During this period the fashion of wearing wigs enabled the wealthy, who alone could afford to buy them, to use hair as a badge of status and riches. In Germany, during the Wartburg Festival in 1817, revolutionary students ceremonially committed the powdered wig to the flames, as a symbol of the old regime. Earlier, during the French Revolution, heads and wigs rolled as the guillotine fell, and it would be satisfying to record that the new citizen leaders eschewed all the old vanities. Unfortunately, this is not quite true. Hair styles from then on were certainly modified, and not only in France, but the new elite was easily distinguishable from the rank and

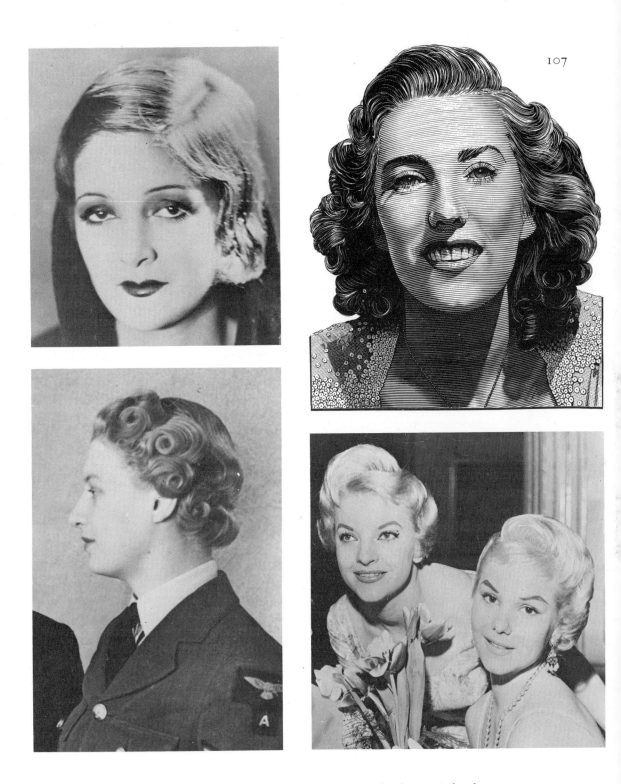

World War II produced in England short hair styles that were supposed to be practical and easy to manage, but that were not markedly different from those of the 1930s (top left). The women's services insisted on hair being cut short above the collar (bottom left) but longer hair was still favored by entertainers who had to supply glamor even in the midst of austerity—such as Britain's "forces favorite" Vera Lynn (top right). By the 1950s styles had become more varied and women had begun to experiment with the new hair colorants (bottom right).

file. Pictures of Mirabeau, Lafayette, and Robespierre show them with at least the appearance of fashion and wealth, contrasting with revolutionaries who stemmed from the people, such as the brewer Santerre, or the cobbler Simon, who guarded Louis XVII in prison.

The English Civil War offers the clearest example of hair being used as a political banner. The long hair of King Charles I and his followers proclaimed the Royalist party. Not all Parliamentarians wore short hair with their plain clothes and white collars. Indeed, once again, leaders such as Cromwell, Ireton, and Fairfax wore their hair long. But the fanatic Puritans within the party made short hair a matter of principle, and so the Roundhead legend grew. Again, it was a case of both reaction and assertion. Short hair and simple clothes were a reaction against the luxurious fashions of king and court. But they were also the age-old assertion of purity, a turning away from sex and worldliness, combined unhappily with the age-old intolerance and lack of charity that has so often marred such ideals. Thus, with the return of Charles II to London in 1660, fine clothes and fine wigs again became the badges and banners of a permissive age.

It becomes more difficult to theorize about hair styles when we go further back in time. Take the Middle Ages in Europe. The early part was a frankly sexual age. Men mostly wore their hair long and many wore beards. The hair of young girls was usually long and loose, and plaited or braided in older women. Nudity was no cause for shame: women raised their skirts deliberately as a mark of honor to great men.

The Church grafted its moral codes, its sexual taboos, its dogma of celibacy, and its disapproval of long hair and beards onto this medieval sexuality. It was the beginning of a long struggle for body and soul, and the beginning of a sort of sexual neurosis involving perversions, sodomy, flagellation, and hysteria. It is noticeable that hair was worn shorter by the end of the 13th century and shaving was much more common, though this may have been due as much to the new availability of soap as to the efforts of the Church. Perhaps the worst effect of these sexual obsessions of the Church was on women. As the source of all sexual evil and objects of contamination, their whole status became degraded. Because their hair was considered provocative, it must be hidden, and as the early Church believed that the Virgin Mary had conceived through the ear, female ears had to be hidden too. The result was the wimple, which was designed to give a chaste appearance, but which women rapidly adapted into a charming fashion, entirely defeating its purpose. Hairlessness became something of a fetish for women. Head hair was not only concealed but shaved or plucked to give an artificially heightened forehead, and eyebrows were removed too.

Opposite, the studied, expensively achieved casualness of the hair style of one of today's international motion-picture beauties, Catherine Deneuve. Overleaf: by contrast Paul Gauguin (1848–1903) painted a Tahitian girl whose head—and body—hair owed nothing to the attentions of the cosmetician or hairdresser.

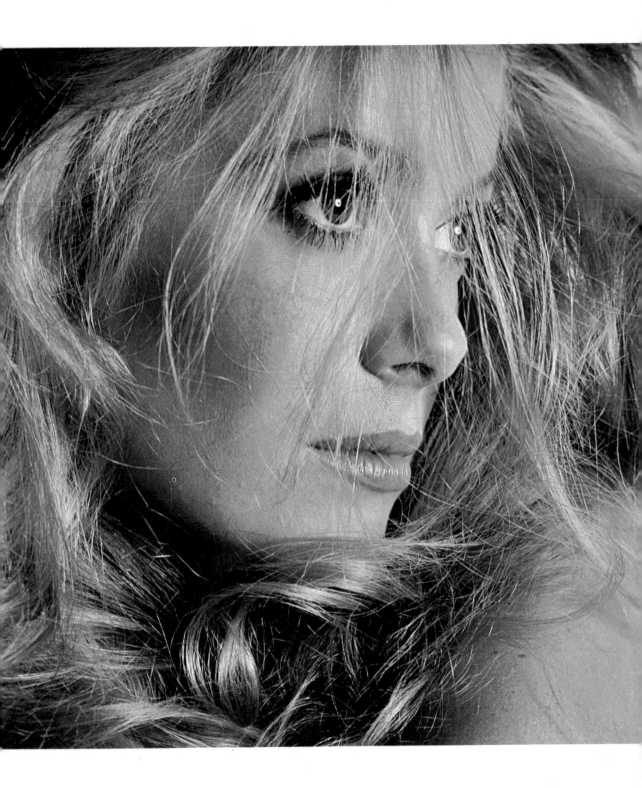

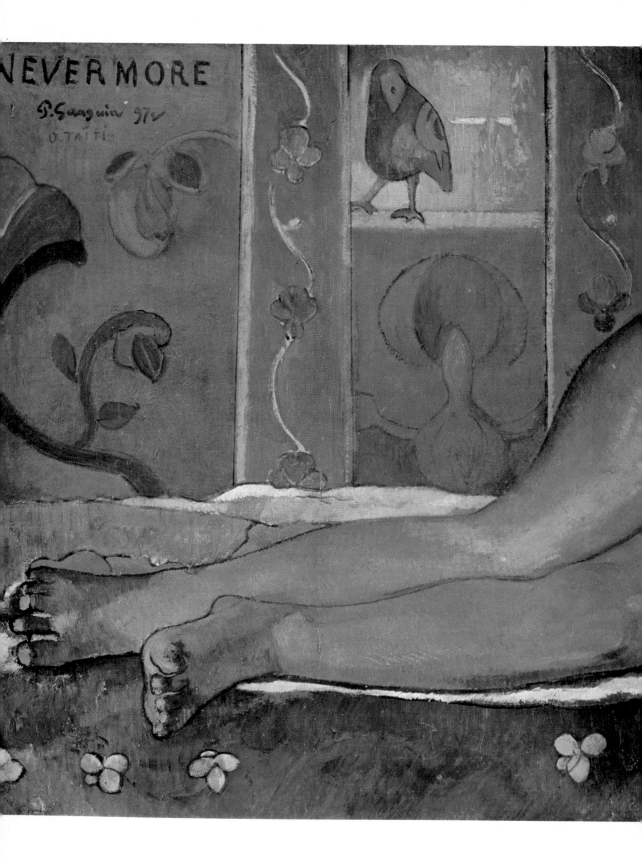

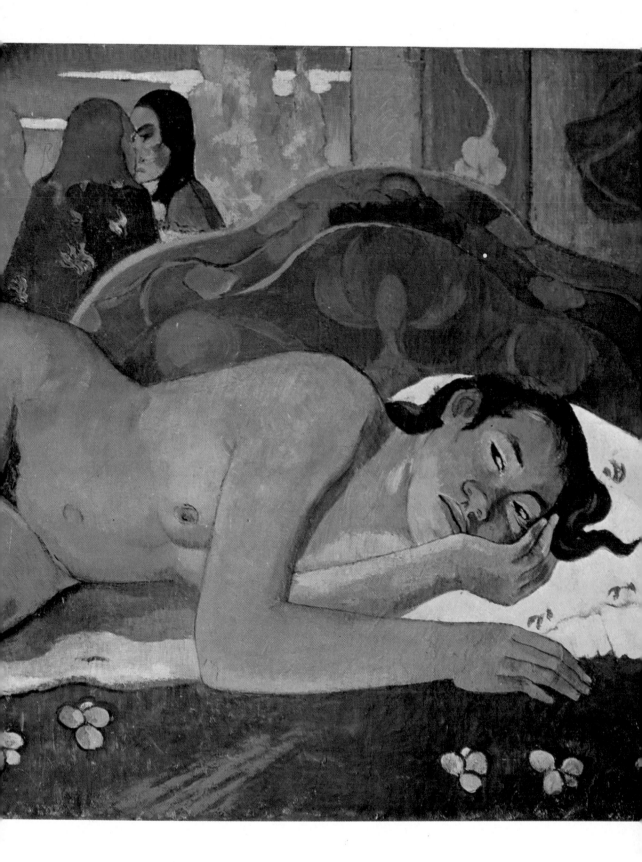

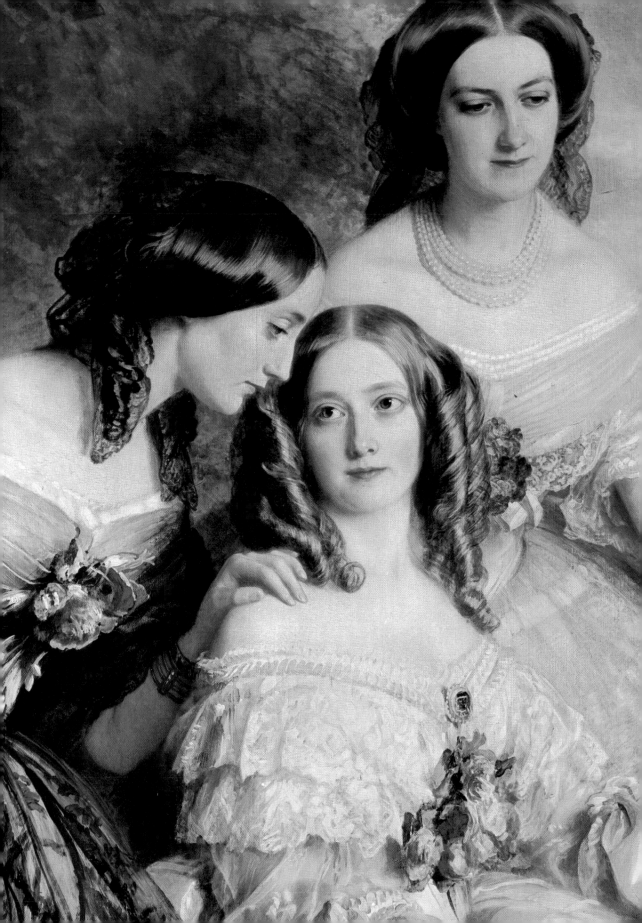

In this chapter, we have concentrated closely on sophisticated societies, but hair styles play a part also in primitive cultures, where, however, they tend to be a male prerogative. In *The Mothers* (1927), Robert Briffault described how, in a number of East African tribes, it was the men who indulged in luxurious costumes and hair styles. The Acholi, for example, wore a cone of matted hair into which were interwoven beads, ostrich and parrot feathers, shells, brass cartridge cases, and pieces of ivory, whereas the women simply plaited their hair. Among the Dodingo and Tulondo, elaborate bowl-shaped headdresses ornamented with shells were worn by the men, but the women's heads were completely shaven. The Mashukulumba male rivaled the English Macaroni of the 18th century, for Briffault described his tapering headdress as sometimes a yard long. A woman of this tribe not only shaved her own hair, but was expected to present it to her future husband to help pad out his extravagant coiffure.

Throughout the world, primitive costumes and hair styles have been undermined by constant exposure to the cultural and commercial pressures of the white man. The 17th-century Dutch mariner Abel Tasman, and James Cook, the English explorer of the following century, described the original hair style of the Maoris of New Zealand as a topknot ornamented with up to three white feathers, or with combs. By 1830 the missionaries who followed in the wake of the pioneer explorers had had such influence that many natives were cutting their hair short. Today, the Maoris adopt western hair styles and copy film stars. Nevertheless, traditional styles still survive in less exposed areas. In the villages and kraals of Africa, tribal custom in both dress and hair style have persisted, and it is the men who still steal the show. In *Women of Africa* (1960), Alastair Scobie writes:

"Everything a woman does to her hair is demure beside the tossing lion manes and ostrich plumes, the proud black feathers and ochred elegance of the warriors. Perhaps the men of the Suk of Northern Kenya have the oddest hair style of all. From a hard shell of hair stiffened with brilliantly colored clay (often white and purple if I remember right), a long, curving wire holds a bobble above the head.

"Unfortunately for the women of Africa, the black crinkled hair will seldom make an interesting hair style. The Swazi women of South Africa wear it long, caught in a bushy mass that is not unattractive. Zulu women wear their hair piled high and fixed with red clay into a shape like a seventeenth-century top hat without the brim. The Ndebele women (kin to the Swazi and Zulu) seem to shave their heads for preference."

Among the primitive Indian tribes of South America, once again it is the men's hair styles that are particularly elaborate. Most pluck their facial

Opposite: the Empress Eugénie, wife of Napoleon III of France, with her ladies of honor: the smooth top, center part, and ringlets are not intended to seem anything but what they are—a creation of the hairdresser's skill.

hair, but allow head hair to grow to around shoulder length. The Jivaros, probably the largest tribe in northern South America, and famous for their unpleasant habit of head-shrinking, are hypersensitive about their glossy black hair. It is cut straight across the forehead, but allowed to grow to waist length at the back. The tribe can be identified by the three pigtails the men wear—a long one behind and a short one on each side. In addition, they wear a belt of human hair. The most colorful hair style among South American Indians must be that of the Colorado Indians— one of only two tribes to survive in the jungle retreats of the Ecuadorean lowlands. They paint both bodies and hair bright red.

In neither primitive nor sophisticated societies have fashions in body hair been so varied or extravagant as those for head hair. In sophisticated communities, except in intimate circumstances, most body hair is concealed by clothing, so there has never been the same pressure to follow or compete with styles set by fashion leaders. In fact, fashions in body hair seem to be a question of cultural conditioning, with personal preferences and sexual inclinations taking over in individual cases. It seems to be the one case in which women are prepared to please men, yielding to masculine whims and demands, even when in the past this has meant depilation by quite painful methods. This is in strong contrast to women's usual indifference to men's clearly expressed preferences regarding head hair. Men plead and scold in repeated efforts to get women to wear their hair long and loose, but if current fashion dictates otherwise, as it most often does, male wishes are totally ignored. On the other hand, if a lover shows a preference for body hair to be shaved, then it usually is. In this more direct sexual context, the old pattern of submission and dominance between the sexes seems to have been preserved.

This may well have been the case simply because there has been little high fashion in body hair to offer much of a challenge. There is not, after all, a great deal to be done with tufts of short, coarse, and usually curly hair. The choice has most often been simply between leaving it on or taking it off.

In the Middle Ages, returning Crusaders brought back the Arabic idea of depilation for women, and for a time it was adopted by the European aristocracy. In *The French Art of Sex Manners,* Georges Valensin claims that this was terminated by Catherine de Medici, and from then on depilation was practiced only by doctors on hysterical women, as a means of making the "suffocating humors of the brain flow to a place that was quick to receive them." A report by a certain Jean de la Montagne from Lyons in 1525 stated that it was considered elegant then to be completely shaven.

Right, a young Pialla tribesman from New Guinea; his wig is made from the hair of a dead relative woven on a bamboo frame. Far right, some African hair styles as seen by a European traveler in the 19th century.

Court ladies had superfluous hair removed from the lower as well as the upper half of their bodies. Twenty years later, however, according to a contemporary historian, they applied a special pomade to their private parts to make the hair grow abnormally long, so that it could be "curled like a Saracen's moustache" and ornamented with colored bows.

Depilation had been the fashion, of course, in ancient Egypt, Greece, and Rome. Even King Solomon is reputed to have demanded that the Queen of Sheba remove "nature's veil" before he would sleep with her. But neither our cultural inheritance from Greece and Rome nor the brief influence of the harem-haunted Crusaders appears to have had much long-term effect in Britain, or subsequently in America. Although shaving of axillary hair in women has been more popular, shaving of pubic hair seems to have been a minority practice. In fact some 19th-century euphemisms for pubic hair, such as "Cupid's arbor" and "grove of Eglantine," are charming enough to suggest quite a positive appreciation, although an 18th-century one, "parsley," is less flattering in its down-to-earth agricultural flavor. Perhaps the clearest indication of pubic hair having been both fashionable and desirable is the existence of pubic hair wigs. These were popular in England in the 17th century and were called "merkins." The 19th-century term was a "bowser," and this device enjoyed a renewed popularity in the present century. According to the Italian novelist C. Malaparte, in *The Skin* (1952), during and just after

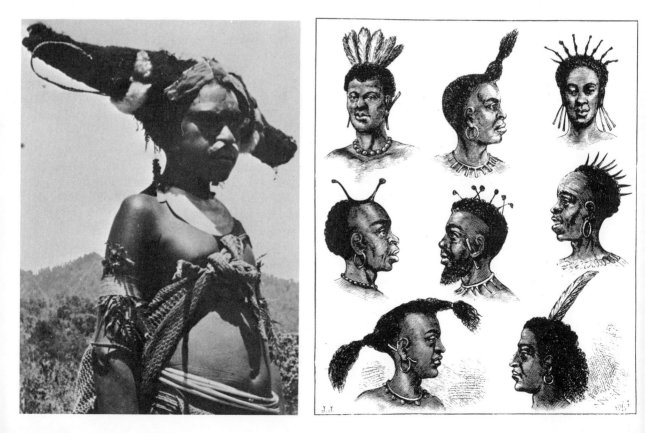

World War II, Neapolitan prostitutes not only bleached their pubic hair, but also wore merkins, to provide the blondeness required by some soldier clients. Pubic wigs are still obtainable today from certain hairdressers in most of the larger cities of the Western world. But it is as well to see these oddities in perspective. They find their way into the records of any period simply because they are amusing, but they represent the fringe behavior of a minority.

All the same, there is some significance in the fact that the permissive society has bestowed its blessing on pubic hair both as a topic of conversation and as a new fashion feature. In England, the fashion designer Mary Quant earned the title of first modern leader in pubic hair fashion, with her statement: "We shall move towards exposure and body cosmetics, and certainly pubic hair—which we can now view in the cinema and on the stage—will become a fashion emphasis, although not necessarily blatant. I think it is a very pretty part of the female anatomy; my husband once cut mine into a heart shape; pubic hair is almost aesthetically beautiful, anyway. Women are incredibly well-designed streamlined creatures and should be seen more." In America, Lillian Roxon, a journalist authority on the wild world of the young, stated in New York, in a special interview for the London *Sunday Mirror:* "In the seventies women will stop shaving their body hair. By 1975 every pretty girl will have hairy legs. Otherwise she will look old-fashioned."

The survey on attitudes to body hair carried out for this book at a British university certainly confirms some increased interest among the young in pubic hair. A number of girls thought women had to pay attention to it these days, and a midwife stated that she had noticed that the pubic hair of women in hospital now shows evidence of care. Two girls thought that fashion would shortly demand that women show their pubic hair, and one housewife, who believed that there was no increase in interest, was surprisingly found to be an early follower of Mary Quant, for she sported a "pubic heart." However, only 12 per cent of the girls interviewed confessed to shaving or trimming their pubic hair. Far more, some 98 per cent, shaved axillary hair or removed it with depilatory creams, and of the three girls who failed to do this, two were yielding to the special request of their boyfriends. In 50 per cent of the cases, aesthetic as well as hygienic reasons were given for the fashion.

We have already seen in the previous chapter that art, for a variety of reasons, has failed to record fashions in body hair accurately, and the British journalist and author Kenneth Allsop, in an amusing article, "The Great Pubic Hair Controversy," that appeared recently in the London

In most of the Western world today women remove—mostly by shaving—their underarm hair (far right) and the hair of their legs (right). In this they seem willing to yield to male preference, as they do not where head hair is concerned. Perhaps this is simply because, while head hair is often on public display, body hair is a more private and intimate possession.

magazine *Nova,* commented: "Art itself (what might be called public art, that is other than pornographic or deliberately erotic) has been interestingly ambiguous about the natural furriness of the human body. The Greeks, 400 B.C., were carefully chipping out the curly fleece in marble, whereas the Romans (a prudish suburban lot who were shocked by the nakedness of Greek athletes) left the area smooth. But that was on male statues. When they did portray girls they were almost mathematical exercises, as in the Esquiline Venus, with a plump but hairless curve. Henceforth it gets more confused. Some Florentine painters, such as Da Sento, put in the hair; Titian's Venus had a seven o'clock shadow, Giorgione's model apparently used depilatory cream. After Christian morality had devalued the classical ideal of the body as emblem of divine perfection, nudes were seen morose with shame ('They knew that they were naked'): hands, foliage or draperies shielding the centres of carnal lust. In the Low Countries hair began to creep back in, as a dusky suggestion in Van Eyck and Dürer, and most distinctly with the post-Reformation enjoyment of pin-up nudity as supplied by Cranach. The most curious inconsistency is in the modern period. When Cézanne or Bonhomme or Delvaux or Van Dongen painted in pubic hair there was nothing equivocally coy about it: it was crisp and

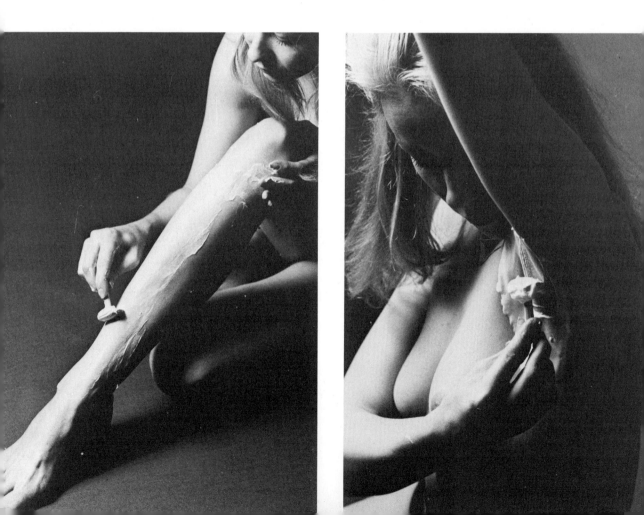

profuse as gorse bushes. Yet simultaneously Degas and Matisse and even Picasso were inserting pink v's, sexless as wedges of processed cheese."

Art has been considerably more helpful when it comes to eyebrows. Medieval and Elizabethan portraits reveal clearly the fashion for plucked eyebrows, which, together with a shaved hairline, gave a uniformly egg-like appearance. Later pictures of fashionable families of the 17th and 18th centuries show permanently surprised faces under heavy brows, obtained by shaving off the natural eyebrows and replacing them with false ones, often made of mouse-skin. By the end of the 18th century, false eyebrows were out and natural ones were merely blackened with a lead comb or brushed with a solution of green vitriol and gum arabic. Later, eyebrow pencils came in, and for a time in the 1920s the natural line was lost again in favor of exaggerated high-shaped brows.

Both the eyebrow and body hair fashions of our relatively advanced societies are curiously reproduced among primitive tribes. Depilation is common among North American Indians, who have sparse body hair anyway, and Andrea Bayard, in her book *Brazilian Eden* (1961), comments: "The Brazilian Indians have no eyebrows or eyelashes. They pluck them out with tweezers shaped from split bamboo. In fact the Indians are absolutely hairless except for the hair on their head, which they keep only because of protection from the sun. Hair on any other part of the body is considered ugly."

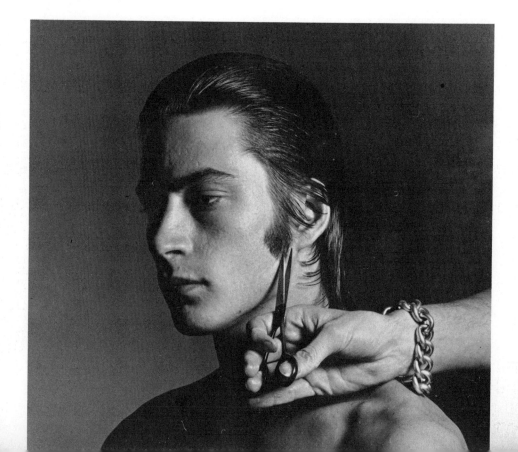

In the South Pacific those old familiars, the Trobriand Islanders, were also great depilators, but the Samoans, although removing armpit hair, very much admired female pubic hair, and a virgin's pubic hair was oiled and combed. African tribes also had cultural fashions for body hair. Among the Bakitara of central Africa, a young girl approaching marriage had all her body hair shaved off, excluding her pubic hair, which was plucked out by her mother. The process was so painful that it took a week to accomplish. The Ba-ila of Northern Rhodesia also required young adults to remove pubic and armpit hair by rubbing it with warm ashes and then plucking.

But in no society has body hair received the same fashionable attention as head hair. The reasons are fairly obvious. The limited areas of body hair give little scope for imaginative or complicated ornamentation, and they are, in any case, often covered by clothing. The head is very different. It is a display point. Varying lengths, tortured shapes, and bizarre styles of both natural and false hair are visual signals. Just as surely as an arrangement of flags on a ship has meaning, so does an arrangement of hair speak in its own coded language. In every age and in almost every culture, hair or wigs have been used to denote status and to serve as a badge or, sometimes, as a disguise.

In the 1970s men have broken away from their long subjection to crewcut conformity. It is no longer thought effeminate for a man to have a hair style created for him (left). Nor is it any longer possible to distinguish between specifically male and specifically female hair styles (below).

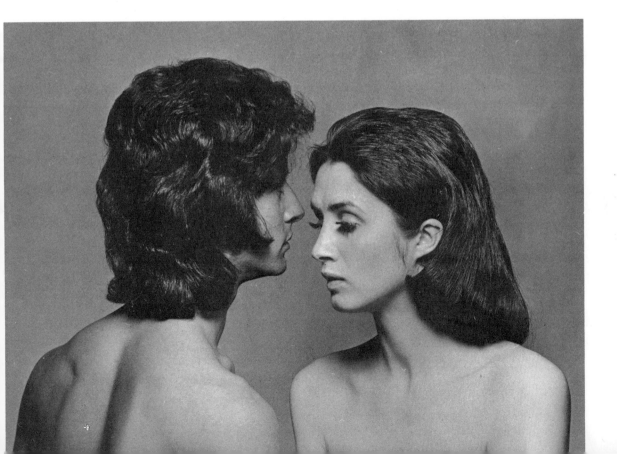

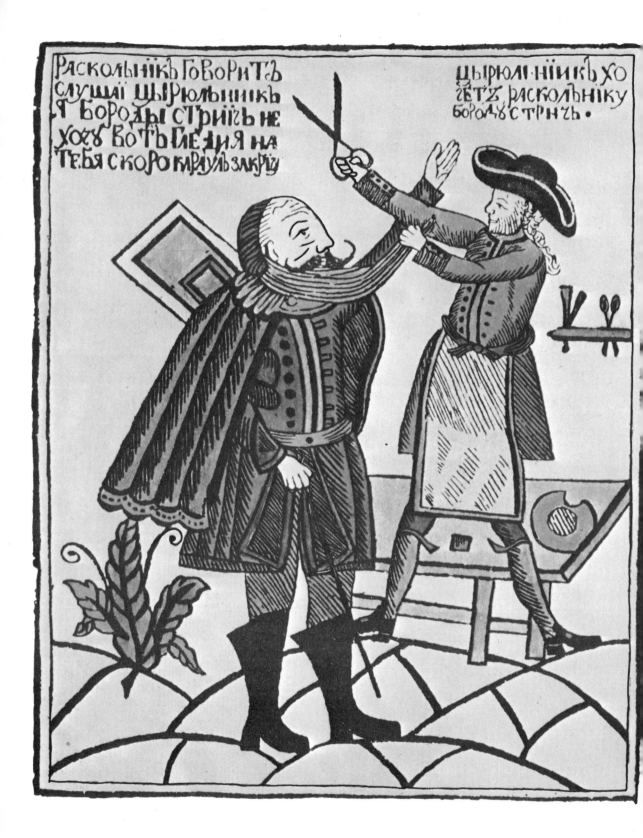

5 *Wigs, Badges, and Disguises*

Wigs have kept appearing in these pages, as they have on heads throughout history, and their very persistence must earn them consideration in their own right. Even more than natural hair, wigs have been used both as badges and disguises. First and foremost they have served, just as natural hair styles often have, as badges of the elite. In Europe and America they have also served, particularly during the 17th and 18th centuries, as badges of different professions. Even today, in England, barristers and judges still wear their distinctive wigs, and the tradition lingers on in Black African countries, such as Kenya and Ghana, which once knew British rule. As disguises, wigs have a long theatrical history, from Greek drama, through the Elizabethan theatre, to the drag shows of today.

It all began at least as far back as ancient Egypt, with something of a democratic touch, for wigs then were worn by everyone except laborers and priests. All the same, the badge still worked, for the richer the owner, the richer and more ornate the wig. The finest wigs were normally made of human hair, although more extravagant materials were occasionally used. One wig discovered with a mummy from the 26th dynasty (about 600 B.C.) was made of pure silver. Wigs of fabulous cost were interred with the wealthy dead, to act as symbols of affluence and importance even beyond the grave.

There are records of wigs being worn by Assyrians, Persians, Phoenicians, Lydians, Carians, and of course the Greeks and Romans. In Greece, wigs were often crowned with wreaths of flowers, and by the wealthy with diadems of silver and gold. The great Carthaginian general Hannibal (247–183 B.C.) is credited with having two sorts of wigs—one to improve his appearance and the other to disguise himself in battle. In Rome at some

A contemporary woodcut of a barber cutting off the beard of a Russian nobleman in the time of Peter the Great (1682–1725). Peter tried to suppress beards as part of his policy of westernizing Russia.

periods, wigs were such an important item of fashion that portrait busts had removable stone wigs, like lids, so that they could be kept up to date with the changing styles.

Knowing the Roman preoccupation with law and order, it is not surprising to find that prostitutes were not only licensed and taxed, but compelled to display a badge of their profession. They had either to wear a yellow wig, or to dye their own hair yellow. This must have caused some confusion during those periods when virtuous Roman matrons decided that yellow was the fashionable hair color. The Empress Faustina the Elder in the second century A.D. showed more versatility; she was reputed to own several hundred wigs of different colors. An earlier empress, the

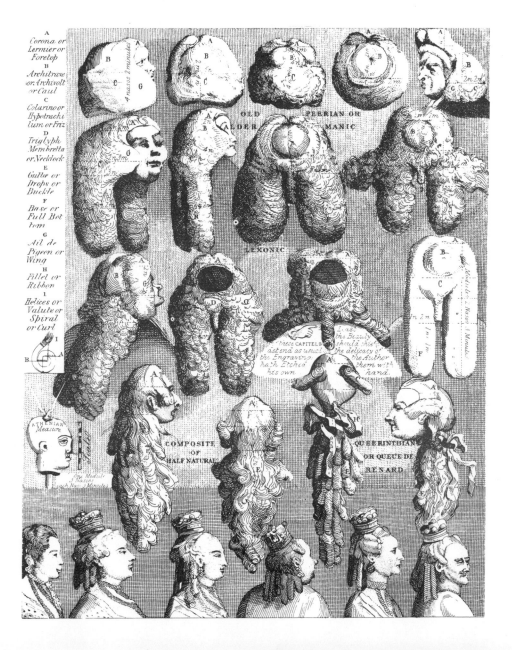

notorious Messalina, used to wear a yellow wig on her nocturnal excursions to brothels. It could not have been very effective as a disguise. When she arrived home without it, as she often did, it was invariably and unerringly returned to her at the palace.

In the Middle Ages in Europe wigs were not much in evidence, but when they were, the Church thundered against them. In the Church's eyes, as we saw in the last chapter, wigs were the badge of the devil. All the same, by the 15th century they were being worn occasionally by men of fashion, mostly to conceal a lack of natural hair. In 1529, during the reign of Henry VIII, the English royal treasury made an official purchase of a wig, but it was not for the king or any of his six wives. It was "a perwyke for Sexton, the king's fool," costing 20 shillings. By 1558, the beginning of Elizabeth's reign, wigs had become an indispensable part of a lady's wardrobe and were worn also by some men. Women's wigs were often dyed red as a compliment to the queen, who had had natural red hair in her youth. She herself owned at least 80 wigs.

The great age of wigs for men began in France, when Louis XIII took to wearing a periwig in 1624. It could have been considered a disguise, for he had gone prematurely bald at the age of 23, but as taken up by the court and subsequently developed in size and extravagance, it became a badge of wealth. Its use became rapidly de rigueur, but Louis XIV, who came to the throne in 1643, was so proud of his own fair hair that he resisted wearing a wig until after 1670, when he was in his thirties and his hair had begun to thin. As a compliment to the Sun King all his courtiers wore yellow wigs. Later, in old age, Louis took to wearing an enormous wig, thickly covered with perfumed white powder, and at once this practice too was copied by the whole Versailles court, young and old, men and women. A tactful lady-in-waiting was forced to explain to a somewhat disconcerted foreign ambassador: "Everyone wants to look old, for that is to appear to be wise." During the 18th century the Versailles mode for powdered wigs set the fashion for the Western world. By the time he became completely bald, Louis XIV considered the wig so vital to his royal dignity that he never allowed himself to be seen without it by anyone except Binette, his personal barber. It was passed to him through the curtains of his four-poster bed. There is no record of whether he kept it on in bed for the benefit of his many mistresses, or whether the royal nightcap was considered sufficient camouflage.

Charles II of England, who had been in exile at Versailles, brought the fashion to his own country. He took to a wig when his own dark hair began to turn gray. After his Restoration in 1660, periwigs became a

A satirical engraving by William Hogarth (1697–1764) mocks some of the more extravagant periwigs available during the golden age of the wig in England.

positive mania in English society. They grew in size to absurd dimensions. An elaborate full-bottomed wig could cost as much as £200, although the diarist Samuel Pepys records buying a fine one for £4 10s. and later two more for £3 and £2. Even inventories of clothes for English schoolboys to take to boarding school included periwigs, and from the age of six, when they ceased to dress like girls, most well-to-do boys were made to wear wigs for Sundays and great occasions. Prices varied from only 16 shillings to many guineas, with a regular outlay of two shillings or so for half a pound of hair powder each week. A small linen cap was worn between the wig and the head to absorb perspiration.

The difficulty of keeping natural hair clean added to the convenience of wigs. Pepys was at first in two minds about them, but in 1665, while a wig was being repaired, became converted. "This day," he wrote, "after I had suffered my owne hayre to grow long, in order to wearing it, I find the convenience of periwiggs is so great that I have cut off all short again and will keep to periwiggs."

Needless to say, North America was not left behind. Despite protests from Puritan ministers like the famous Increase Mather, who was also an author and President of Harvard University, the fashion spread. Mather denounced wigs as "horrid bushes of vanity," but his son Cotton, also a well-known clergyman and author, adopted the style, along with most of the clergy. In the South the fashion was general, not only among wealthy planters and gentlemen but among blacksmiths, innkeepers, and bricklayers. Slaves, who could not afford even secondhand wigs, contrived strange copies from cottonwool and goat-hair.

As the elite introduced more and more extravagant styles to keep ahead of the masses, professional groups became identified with special shapes. The British writer James Stewart in his *Plocacosmos* (1728) refers to "the clerical, the physical [for doctors], and the tie peruke for the man of the law, the brigadier or major for the army and navy," and says that "the merchant, the man of business and of letters were distinguished by the grave full-bottom or more moderate tie, neatly curled; the tradesman by the snug bob or natty scratch, the country gentleman by the natural fly and hunting peruke .... All conditions of men were distinguished by the cut of the wig, and none more so than the coachman who wore his, as there does some to this day, in imitation of the curled hair of a water dog."

It was the same in France. In his *Pogonologia* (1786), Jacques Dulaure wrote: "A tradesman . . . to appear as he ought, should have his head shaved and wear a round wig; physicians and surgeons too should do the same. Who, in this enlightened age, would put the least confidence in a

The moustache is often an identifying facial badge that makes the role or personality of its owner instantly recognizable. The 19th-century advertisement for a fixative (center left) shows some of the forms it can be made to take. Top left: the bizarre moustache of Surrealist painter Salvador Dali. Top right, the military moustache—of a sergeant-major in the British army. Center right, the revolutionary moustache, that of Che Guevara. Bottom: German fuhrer Adolf Hitler (left) and comedian Charles Chaplin (right) gave different personalities to the same shape of moustache.

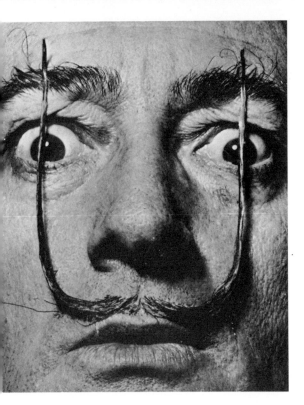

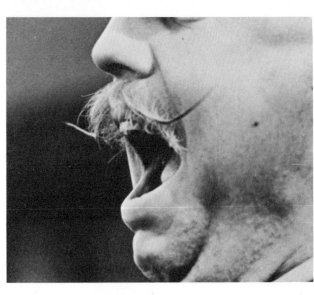

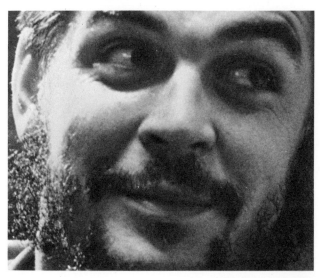

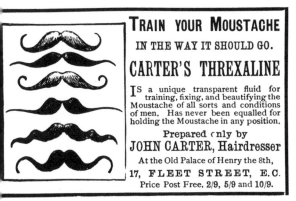

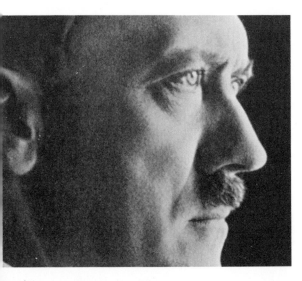

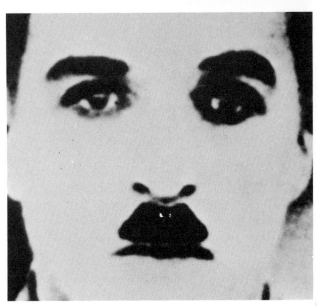

126 physician who wears his own hair, were it the finest in the world? A wig, certainly, can't give him science, but it gives him the appearance, and that is everything nowadays."

So necessary was the authoritative badge of the appropriate wig that in the English periodical *Connoisseur* for April 24, 1755, a certain mode of behavior and dress was condemned because it was as "improper as a physician would seem ridiculous prescribing in a bag-wig, or a serjeant pleading in the Court of Common Pleas in his own hair instead of a night-cap periwig." In the *London Magazine* for 1753 appeared a mock advertisement in which a wig-maker, "Monsieur de la Papillotte," claimed that "to ecclesiastical perriwigs he gives a certain demure air; he confers on the tye-wigs of the law an appearance of great sagacity and deep penetration; on those of the faculty of physick, he casts a solemnity and gravity that seem equal to the profoundest knowledge. His military smarts are mounted in a curious manner, quite unknown to every workman

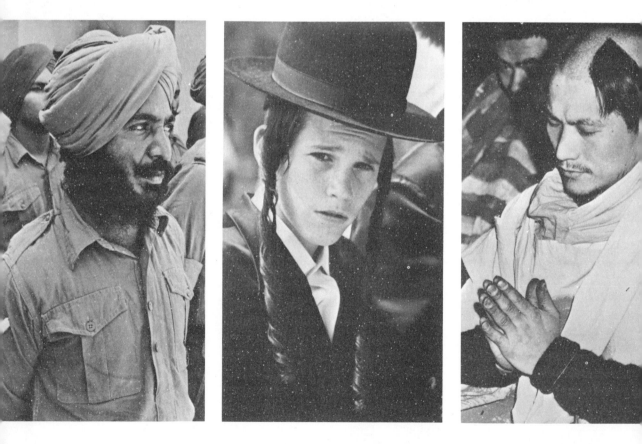

Hair is used almost as much as costume to proclaim religious belief or dedication. Left, a Sikh soldier whose religion forbids him to cut his hair and so over-rules the military convention of short hair. Center, the long, curled side locks of an Orthodox Jewish boy in modern Israel. Right: in 1970 this Vietnamese shaved all except four patches of hair from his head and vowed to remain shaven in this way until the end of the war in Vietnam.

but himself; he throws them into what he calls the animating buckle, which gives the wearer a most warlike fierceness."

In the British army of the mid-18th century, where the Ramillies wig, which had a braided queue, was the favorite of the officers, the habit of wearing wigs spread even to the ranks, and a weekly ration of one pound of flour was issued per soldier for powdering them.

With large wigs so expensive, wig thieves became ingenious. John Gay, the English poet and dramatist, described how they used a covered basket, a tall man, and a small boy:

> Nor is the wig with safety worn;
> High on the shoulder, in a basket born,
> Lurkes the small boy, whose hand to rapine bred,
> Plucks off the curling honours of thy head.

Other wig thieves specialized in robbing passengers in hackney coaches. They would cut an opening in the back of the coach, snatch the passengers' wigs, and disappear into the night. Yet, not long afterward, wigs that had cost sometimes as much as £140 could be bought for six pence in London's street markets.

The death of Louis XIV in 1715 proved to be a death-blow for the full-bottomed wig. Fashion began to favor smaller, less pretentious, and much less costly models. In England, the middle and even the lower classes could now afford to wear wigs. By the 1760s, more and more men were sporting their own hair. In 1765 in London, worried peruke-makers petitioned the king to require men by law to wear wigs. The final eclipse of the wig stemmed indirectly from the French Revolution, which set more than heads rolling. Wigs were associated with the privileges of the *ancien régime* and the reaction against them sealed their fate. Wigs lingered into the 19th century, worn chiefly by old and conservative men, and survived into this century only as trappings of the law, part of ancient pageantry, or to be worn furtively by a few people to disguise the loss or paucity of their natural hair.

And then, in 1958, the hair stylist Carita designed wigs for all Givenchy's models as a gimmick for the Paris fashion shows. They caused a sensation. *Life* magazine took up the story and a new age of wigs was born. The modern wig might well have been, like its predecessors, a badge of wealth. But modern technology, at precisely the right moment, produced convincing synthetic hair, which brought prices tumbling down. So wigs became, at least at first, a badge of the "with-it," trendy set. Worn initially almost as a joke, their convenience soon convinced women they should be taken seriously. The 20th-century woman might not be in Rome while her hair was blushing on the Rhine, but she could be getting on with a busy life while her wig went to the hairdresser. The modern wig so perfectly imitates real hair that a woman can wear it openly as a fashion, or secretly as a disguise. Either way, it has become a positive hazard to Customs and Immigration officers, confronted by a blonde with long, straight hair, whose passport photograph depicts a curly-haired brunette.

Wigs for men, although increasing in popularity, still fall primarily into the category of disguises. There is, however, some indication that they are coming more blatantly into their own. Way-out styles, such as the Afro look, are more easily achieved, even by a Negro, by the use of a wig. In fact, all extreme hair styles tend to favor wigs; people are more inclined to allow the hairdresser to experiment with an unprotesting and expendable wig than with their own more precious hair.

In drama, the use of wigs is greater than it has ever been, not only because of the development in this century of film and television, but because modern insistence on period accuracy for fashions extends to hair styles, and is often best achieved with wigs. The use of wigs to enable male players to impersonate female characters remains, though not to the extent it did when women were not allowed on the stage, and young boys played the female parts. Today, the tradition is maintained in the old-fashioned English pantomime, and, in a greatly altered form, by burlesque representations of women by comedians, and in drag shows.

Not only wigs, but false beards, moustaches, and eyebrows, have been part of character makeup over the centuries. The large black moustachios that the villain can twirl in his moment of triumph, and the small pointed beard of the stage Frenchman, are traditional stereotypes. And in a more restrained form, all of these artificial appendages have been employed in the disguises so frequently used by fictional detectives, and even occasionally by their real-life counterparts.

When false beards were worn in real life by the ancient Egyptians, it was certainly not as a disguise, but as a badge of rank—the higher the status, the longer the beard. An upward-curling beard was reserved for gods. Sometimes false beards of metal, often gold, were worn by kings and occasionally, rather confusingly, by queens also. Not to be outdone, the first-century Roman emperor Caligula also wore a false beard wrought in gold. In 14th-century Spain, false beards were so much in fashion that one man might have several colors and styles to wear for various occasions. There was an element of disguise in these, for, hidden behind them, some men indulged in such questionable behavior that King Peter of Aragon was finally compelled to forbid their use.

Opposite: Saint Catherine of Siena performs the symbolic act of cutting off her hair before dedicating herself to a life of virginity as a Dominican nun. Overleaf: Albrecht Dürer (1471–1528) painted his self-portrait as Jesus Christ and gave himself the long hair with which Jesus is traditionally depicted. On page 131, the shaven heads of Buddhist novices in an Indian monastery.

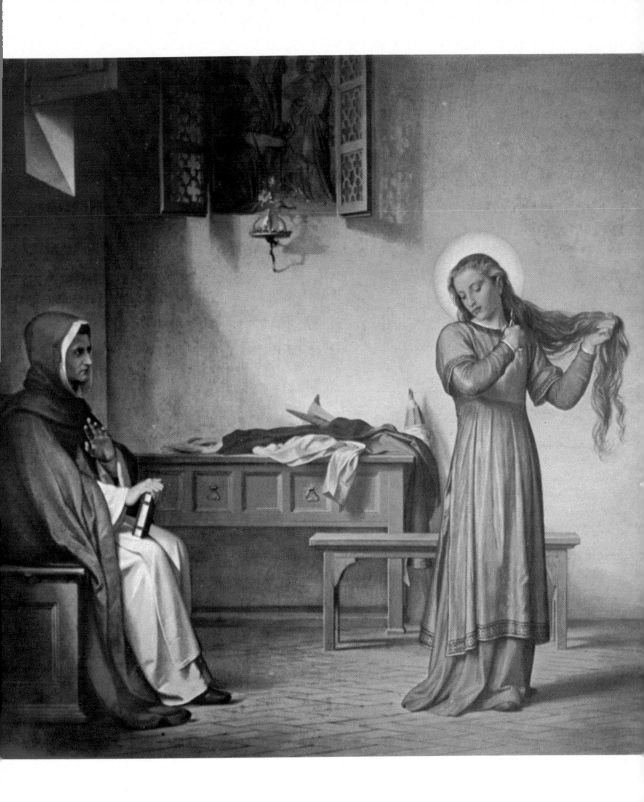

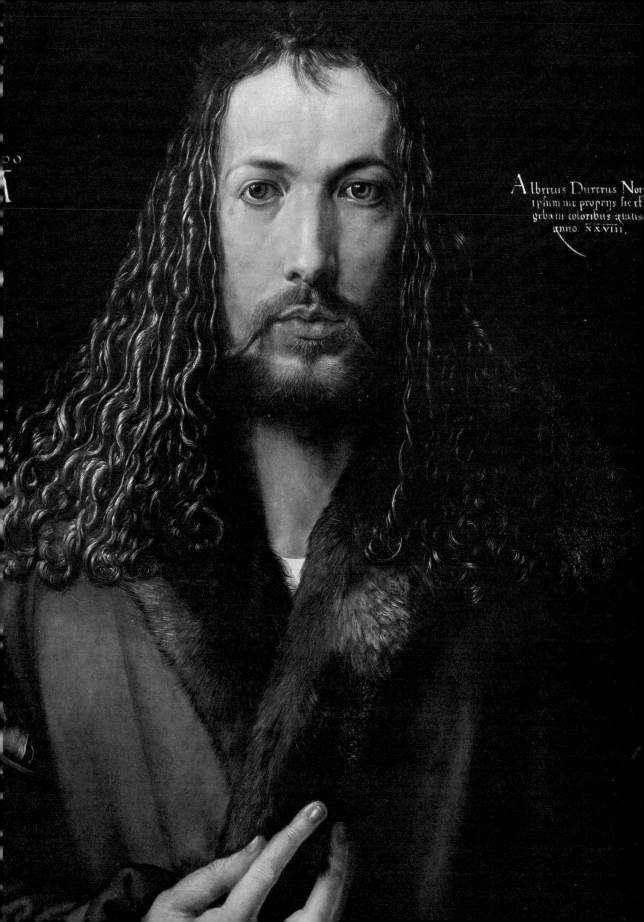

Albertus Durerus Nor
ipsum me proprijs sic ef
gebam coloribus ætatis
anno XXVIII.

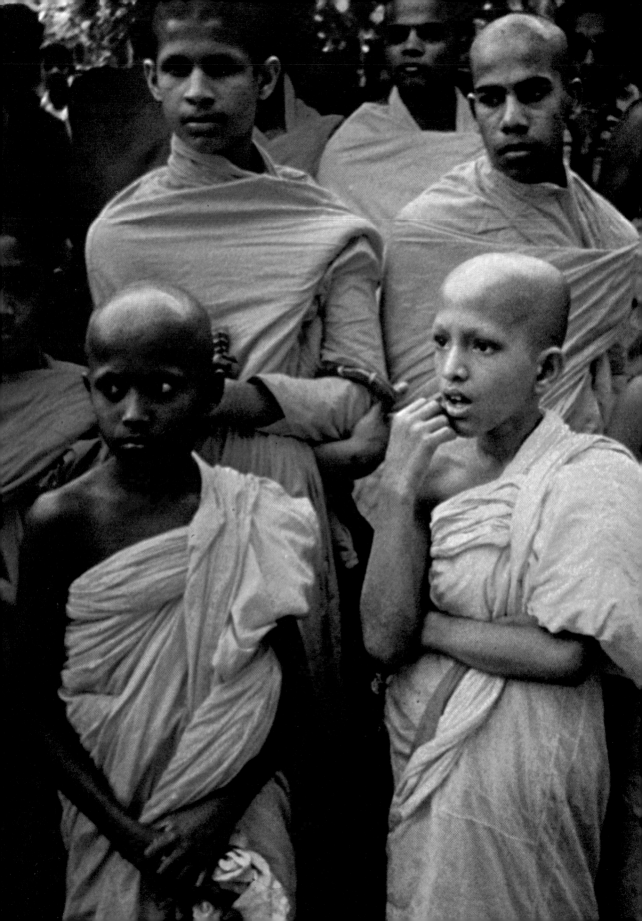

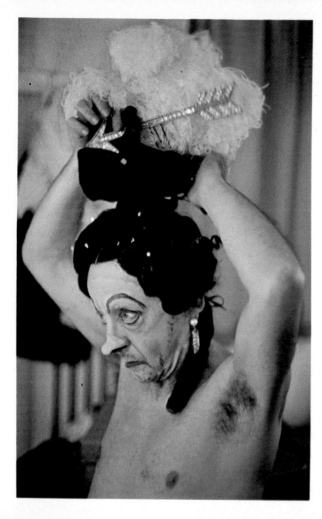
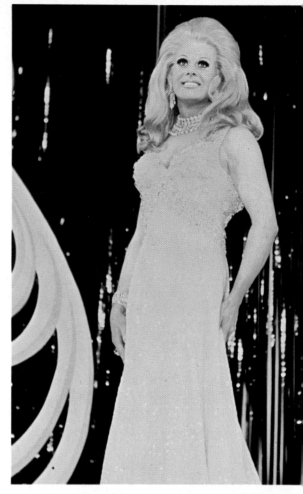
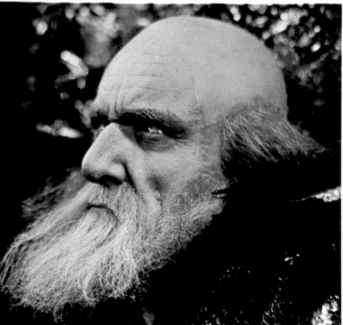
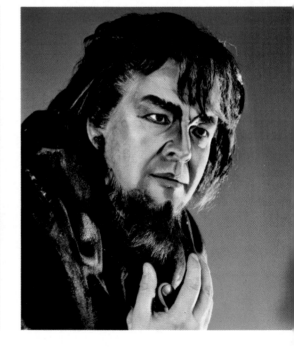

In recent times, false beards seem never to have caught on as a fashion, although in Aldous Huxley's novel *Antic Hay,* published in 1923, the hero, Gumbril, purchases a false beard following a conversation with his tailor, Mr. Bojanus. The latter is convinced that: "The leader has got to look different from the other ones . . . . Some let their 'air grow, like Lloyd George . . . . Some put on black shirts, like this Mussolini, and some put on red ones, like Garibaldi. Some turn up their moustaches, like the German Emperor. Some turn them down, like Clemenceau. Some grow whiskers, like Tirpitz." Gumbril rushes straight to a theatrical wig-maker and buys a fan-shaped beard. "He would, at any rate, be his own leader; he would wear a badge, a symbol of authority."

As with styles in wigs, styles in natural hair have become associated with various social groups. In particular, the way the hair is worn can indicate social, economic, intellectual, or sexual status. In ancient Greece

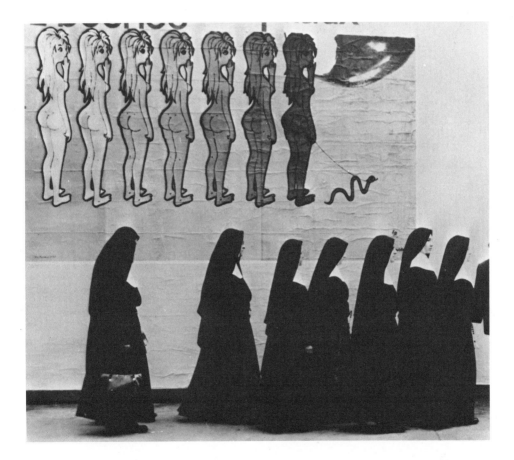

Opposite: hair as disguise in theatrical make-up. Top left, one of the Ugly Sisters in the pantomime Cinderella *adjust "her" wig; top right, a blonde wig is an essential accessory for female impersonator Danny La Rue; bottom left, a bald head and gray beard turns British actor Eric Porter into an aged King Lear; bottom right, the diabolic eyebrows of a stage villain. Above: a contrast in life styles as a group of nuns walks beneath a billboard showing flowing-haired nude girls.*

and Rome, slaves were forced to adopt styles that clearly differentiated them from freemen. Originally they shaved their beards as a mark of servitude. Then, in the third century B.C., when the arrival of Sicilian barbers in Rome started a clean-shaven fashion, they were forced to grow both their hair and beards long, in contrast to their now short-haired and beardless masters. When the Emperor Hadrian reintroduced beards more than three hundred years later, once again the slaves had to shave.

Even during periods in which fashion dictated a clean-shaven chin, beards were retained as the badge of the philosopher. The ancients, in marked contrast to today, revered old age and associated it with wisdom. Because older men and older gods were often dignified by a beard, it followed that other especially wise men should be bearded also. The beard of the Greek philosopher Socrates was so famous that he was described by the Roman satirist Persius, in the first century A.D., as "the Bearded Master." In the same century, the Roman scholar Pliny the Elder spoke of the respect and even fear that was inspired by the beard of the Greek Stoic philosopher Euphrates.

At the time of Peter the Great in Russia a beard was still a badge of wisdom. When one ambassador from the West arrived at the Russian court smooth-cheeked and beardless, Peter protested against the insult. The emissary is reported to have replied: "Had my royal master measured wisdom by the beard, he would have sent a goat." Perhaps this answer made the Czar think again, because some years later he tried to suppress beards in Russia by taxing them.

The whole business of wearing the hair or a beard as a badge is inevitably suspect. A badge simply proclaims what its owner wants people to believe and so it is as likely to be a disguise. A scathing epigram printed in a 17th-century miscellany, *Musarum Deliciae,* edited by Sir John Mennes and J. Smith, makes the point succinctly:

> Thy beard is long, better it would thee fit
> To have a shorter beard and longer wit.

Which really only says what the celebrated Greek orator Herodes Atticus had said in the second century A.D.: "I see the beard and the cloak, but I do not see the philosopher."

In the 19th century, under the influence of the Romantic movement, lofty brows, flowing locks, beards, and whiskers became the badge of the intellectuals and dropouts who opposed the existing social structure. Poets, writers, painters, and bohemians took Victor Hugo, Byron, Baudelaire, and other brilliant men as their models. Once again, there was a danger of affectation. In the Latin Quarter of Paris, the bohemians formed *La*

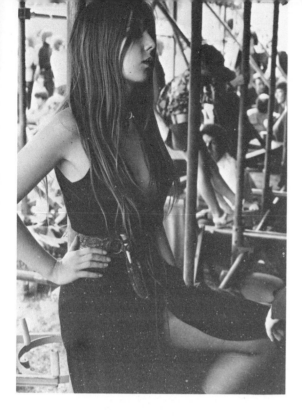

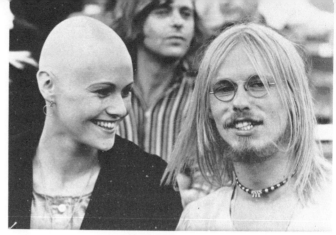

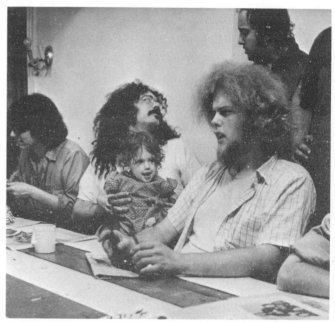

Hippies were immediately recognizable because of their rejection of accepted, conventional hair styles. Their flowing, disheveled hair was in itself a badge of protest. Above, a girl hippy in Paris. Above right, a couple at the Isle of Wight, England, pop festival, 1970—the shaven head of the girl and the straggly hair of the youth are symbols of a deliberate rejection of accepted sexual roles. Right and below, hippies in London. Below right, a US hippy leader whose military-style uniform coat conflicts with the message of peace proclaimed by his long hair.

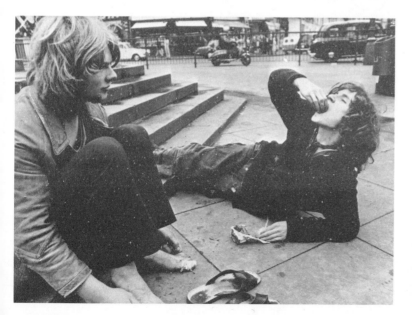

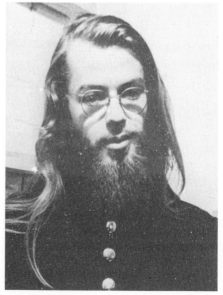

Société des Latifronts, the Association of Noble Brows. In 1834 there were said to be 18 members, and in case nature had not endowed them with a high enough brow, they had an accredited barber at hand to shave the required inch or two of hair above the forehead and produce the lofty aspect to set off their leonine locks. Baudelaire in particular had the reputation of being something of a poseur, acting out alternatively the parts of bohemian and dandy. According to the novelist Champfleury, "One moment his hair would be streaming in elegant, perfumed curls down his neck; the following day his head would be shaved, with a bluish tinge which he owed to the barber's razor." Another contemporary described how: "One day he appeared cleanshaven, like a priest, wore earrings, and even had his hair cropped so that he could wear a blue wig."

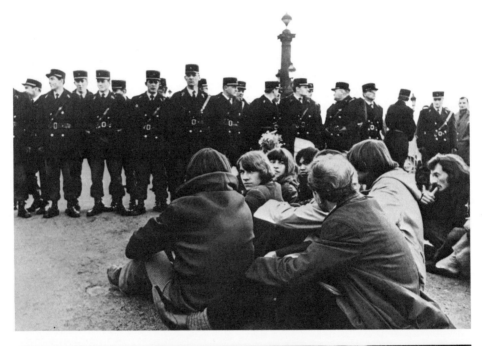

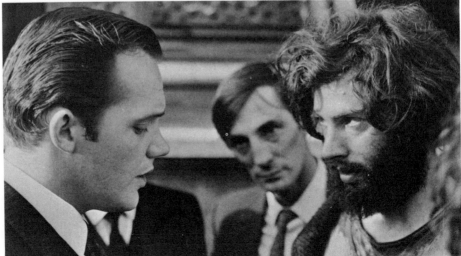

In fact, the image of the long-haired poet, painter, and intellectual has survived right through to this day, though somewhat blurred and overlaid by the popular modern fashion for long hair. A number of protesting groups—not just intellectuals—have adopted the style, from the beats of the fifties, to the more recent rockers, hippies, and Hell's Angels. Today, long hair has become a generalized badge of youth, a symbol of the modern conflict between the generations. It has increasingly proclaimed the rejection of old established values by the young, and their determination to stand out in a deliberately eccentric way from the conformity of the "faceless" and comparatively hairless masses.

This concept of long hair as a symbol of rebellion—although one that can operate effectively only in a predominantly short-haired society—is

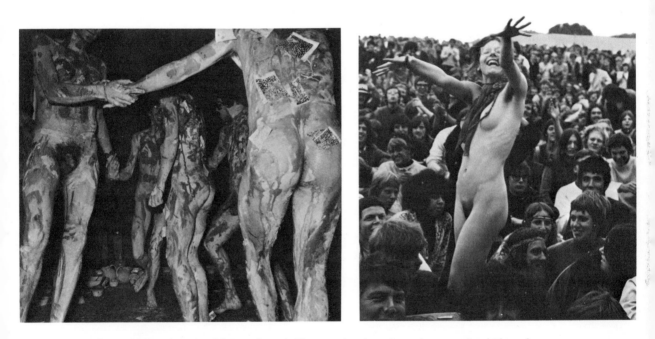

As well as rejecting conventional hair styles, rebellious youth today rejects also conventional ideas of modesty and nudity. They see no reason to be ashamed of the nude body, which they may decorate (above left) or display unadorned (above right). Against this background we may expect rising interest in body hair as a sexual and decorative feature—an interest that is becoming apparent in the refusal of many girls to shave their body hair as their mothers did.

Opposite, top: during the student revolts in Paris in May, 1968, French police—uniformed symbols of authority with conformist, military-type short haircuts—confront a group of students whose long hair as well as their dress proclaims their rebellion. Left, a similar confrontation in London, 1969; a lawyer with a conventional short hair style talks with the disheveled-haired leader of a squatter commune.

made particularly appropriate by the strong association that very short hair has come to have with regimentation, restraint, discipline, and even punishment. The shaved head of the priest, the cropped hair of the prisoner, the crewcut of the American serviceman—all offer the greatest possible contrast to the freedom and individualism expressed in wild, untidy locks. Almost the first order to a new army recruit is likely to be: "Get your hair cut." The modern war machine demands short hair and clean chins. To the ordinary observer, bearded hippies need hardly have bothered to carry their placards, "Make love not war": their hair said it all.

The rebel symbolism of long hair, beards, and sideburns operates at many levels—from the dreamy dropout to the ruthless activist, from the pop singers Bob Dylan and Mick Jagger to the revolutionaries Che Guevara and Fidel Castro. It is ironic that although Marx, Lenin, and Ho Chi Minh all once wore the "rebel" whiskers, as do Castro and Ulbricht today, beards are generally viewed with disfavor in Communist countries. The unkempt look is considered antisocial, and a sign of Western decadence. The Romanian government recently decreed that beards might be grown only by special permission. Acceptable reasons were an acting job, or a scar on the chin. Approved beard owners carry a special license.

Members of a subculture that emerged in Britain in 1967 were faced with a tricky problem. What sort of hair style should they adopt to indicate their rebellion against the rebels? What should they do to

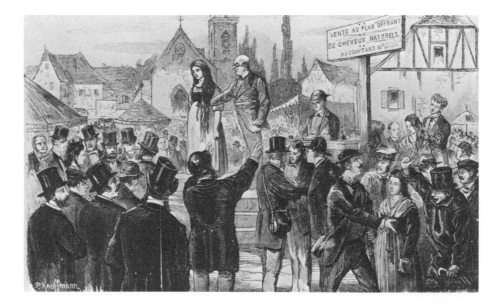

An auction of women's hair in a village in the south of France in the last decades of the 19th century. The hair would have become the wig or hairpiece of a wealthy woman. Today, most wigs are made of artificial fiber, but hair is still bought from Asian peasants for natural hair wigs. In all ages, hair has been sold by the poor for the adornment of the rich.

identify with each other, and yet be distinguished both from the long-haired anti-Establishment and from the Establishment itself? The answer was the singularly unlovely style adopted by the skinheads, who had their hair cut so short that the head looked shaved rather than cropped, and the scalp was clearly visible. Some had the part literally shaved in. Reactionary, racist, with little apparent purpose other than "Paki bashing" (beating up Pakistanis), or putting the boot in (a stomping) when they got the "agro" (aggravation), the skinhead movement was essentially a working-class phenomenon, made up almost exclusively of unskilled teenage manual workers from the poorer urban areas.

Everything about the skinheads was designed to proclaim a defiant pride in their working-class origin—their "braces" or suspenders, worn in preference to belts; their overshort trousers; and their vicious, overlarge

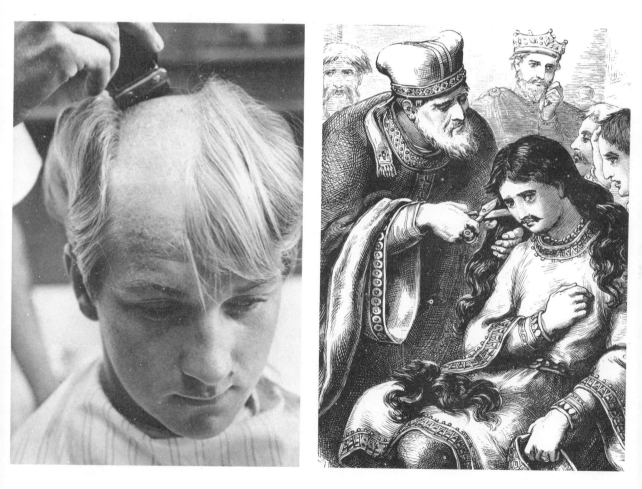

Left, cropping the hair of a recruit to the US Navy, which shares with most military organizations an insistence on short hair as a badge of uniformity and discipline. The Church also has, for different reasons—it saw long hair as a sign of moral laxity—at various periods insisted on men wearing their hair short. Right, Bishop Serlo takes the scissors to lop off a nobleman's locks.

"bovver" boots (bother boots). Even the short hair, easy to keep clean in dirty jobs, fitted the formula. It opposed the opulent locks of the classless, decadent hippies, who, in the skinhead view, "sponged off the state." In contrast, the skinheads adopted an aggressively puritanical image, and in both their cropped heads and attitudes there was a distant echo of the short-haired apprentices who were part of the Puritan scene of Cromwell's day. But these modern "Roundheads" had no politics and no purpose, except bitter retaliation against a hippy youth culture which excluded them and a meritocracy in which they had no merit. They could not drop out because they had never dropped in; they were subliterate rejects, doomed to be unskilled, unqualified laborers. So they banded together and branded themselves "untouchable" with the insignia of their cropped heads.

To find short hair worn with similar bravado as a gauntlet in the face of society, we have to go back to the Reign of Terror in France during the Revolution. Before a woman aristocrat was guillotined she would have her hair cut short over the nape of the neck. This "bobbed" style was imitated by many women, particularly those whose relatives or friends had died on the guillotine. So the new hair style, "à la victime," was a memorial to those who had died and a gesture of contempt to their executioners.

Neither hippy nor skinhead has used the language of hair with quite this precision, nor with the precision that has enabled both natural hair and wigs to be used as a badge not only of class but even of specific trades and occupations. The following passage appeared as late as the 1910 edition of the *Encyclopedia Britannica:* "The footman, whose full-dress livery is the court dress of a hundred years ago, must show no more than the rudimentary whiskers of the early eighteen-hundreds, and butler, coachman, and groom come under the same rule. The jockey and the hunt whip are shaven likewise, but the courier has the whiskers and moustache that once marked him as a foreigner in the English milord's service, and the chauffeur, a servant with no tradition behind him, is often moustached."

Facial hair, as we have seen, has also served as a military badge. In Charlemagne's time, in the confusion of hand-to-hand fighting, it could be a useful distinguishing mark. The emperor, when in battle, is reported to have worn his own long, white, and imposing beard spread over his breastplate, and to have commanded his knights to show their beards in the same way, to distinguish them from the enemy. It is doubtful whether later martial whiskers served half such a useful purpose, but they remained as a military badge. The young man entering an Elizabethan barber's shop could select a beard style that would proclaim him "to be terrible like a warrior . . . ." But in every age these brave, aggressive badges were all too

Periodically throughout history wigs have been worn that make little or no pretence of imitating natural hair. Such wigs are decorations or proclamations in their own right. Top: present-day Afro-style wigs in deliberately non-Afro colors. Bottom left: the gold headdress of a minor wife of Thutmose III of Egypt (15th century B.C.). Bottom right, a modern wig made of steel chain.

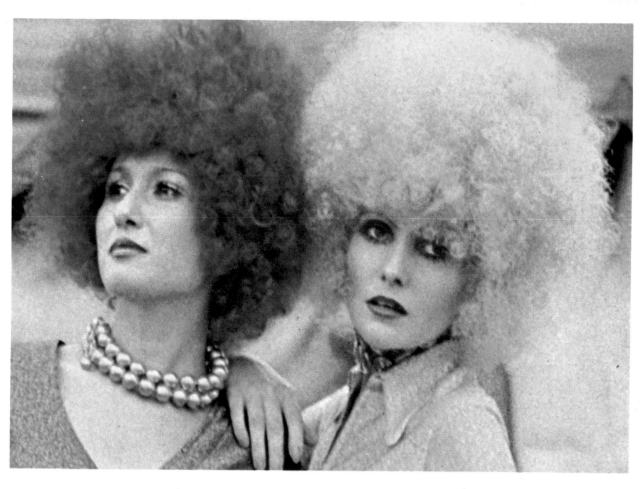

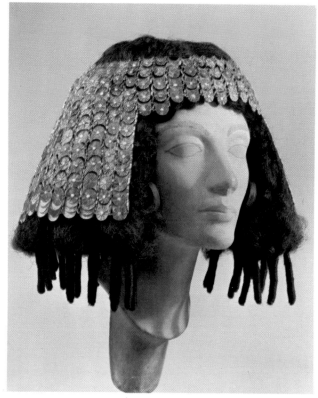

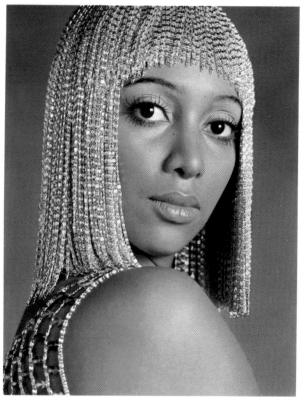

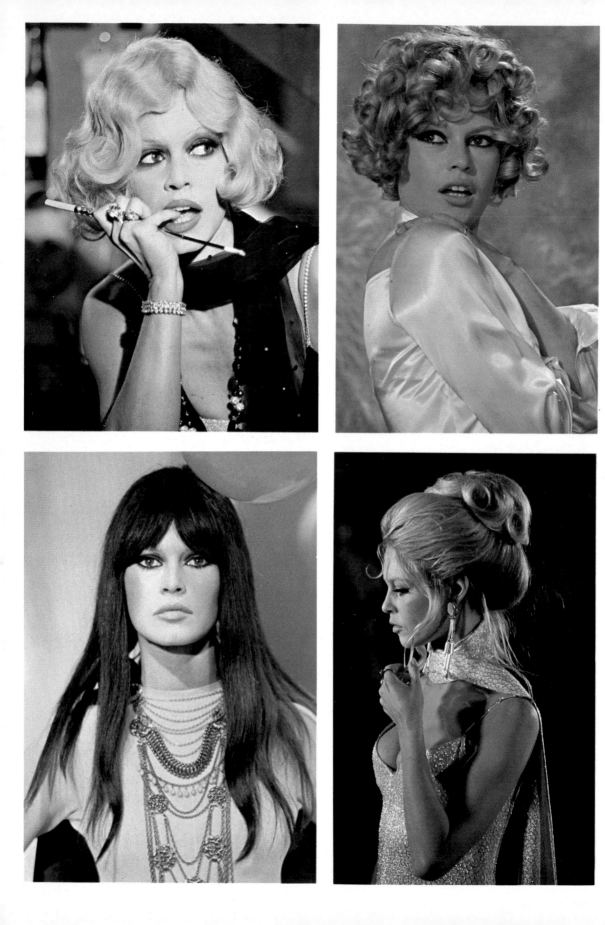

often disguises as well, concealing the loneliness, bewilderment, and fear of ordinary men caught up in the enforced heroics of war.

Statesmen and politicians too have sometimes used hair as a badge and a tool, either to represent the accepted national image or as a deliberate attempt to project their own personalities. The British historian Douglas Johnson has looked at the three leading figures who negotiated the Locarno Pact in 1925, and has suggested that their physical appearance had an important role to play. The success of these discussions seemed vital for the peace of the world, for they marked an attempt to break away from the atmosphere of World War I and to create a new climate of peace between the former antagonists. The major negotiators were Gustav Stresemann of Germany, Austen Chamberlain of Britain, and Aristide Briand of France.

Gustav Stresemann had to contend with hostility at home to the idea of an agreement with the former enemies. It was important that he should represent, both in Germany and abroad, the archetypal German with domed skull and close-cropped hair.

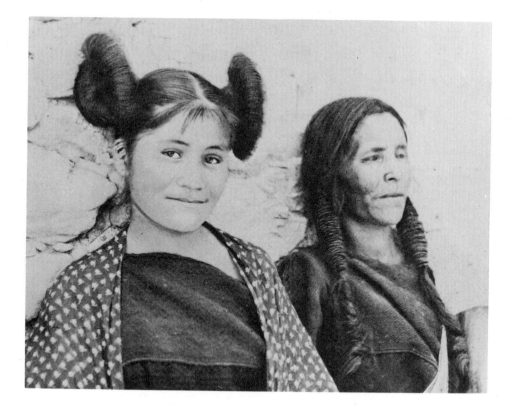

Left: Brigitte Bardot's early popularity was established by her "sex-kitten" image, which included long, carefully casual blonde hair. Simone de Beauvoir wrote of her: "The long, voluptuous tresses of Mélisande flow down to her shoulders, but her hair-do is that of a negligent waif." But these four different wigs give the star four very different images. Above, traditional Eskimo hair styles use hair as a badge of sexual status; the woman on the left is unmarried, when she becomes a wife she also will wear her hair in pigtails.

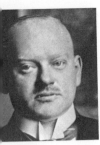

tav Stresemann

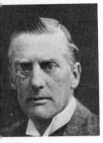

ten Chamberlain

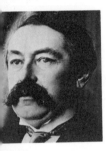

istide Briand

Austen Chamberlain was just as much the accepted image of the Englishman. His hair was neat, sleek, and well-brushed, with perhaps a discreet hint of brilliantine. There was nothing exceptional or eccentric about his appearance and his hair perfectly expressed his nature and his function. Here was someone, it seemed to say, who could be trusted, a gentleman, courteous, unruffled, and affable. In fact, without this very affability, Locarno would never have succeeded.

Aristide Briand of France was in quite a different situation. It was more important for him to project his own image. His extraordinary hair style and moustache proclaimed at once an exceptional man. It marked him out from the ordinary French politician, whom the British and the Germans would automatically distrust, and emphasized the dreamer, the visionary, the famous "pilgrim of peace," who held audiences spellbound as he swore that, for as long as there was breath in his body, he would see that there would be no war. The French themselves were reluctant to sign an agreement with the Germans; perhaps only Aristide Briand could have carried it off; perhaps only someone *looking* like Briand could have succeeded.

Any language is only a convention, a series of accepted shapes imposed on the mouth and larynx to produce sound signals, or on the hair to produce visual signals. From the earliest times this silent language of hair has been used to proclaim sexual status. Once again it has not always been a completely truthful statement. Not every woman whose hair proclaimed her a virgin was one, just as not every tonsured priest was truly celibate. At the most fundamental level, hair that functions as a sexual badge simply differentiates between the sexes to emphasize the male or female role. On a more sophisticated plane, hair can indicate readiness and availability for marriage—not always the same as virginity in cultures where premarital sexual relations have been permitted—or mark out the paired or married woman; or distinguish the widow. It is not surprising that in a largely male-dominated world, in which far stricter standards of sexual behavior have been imposed on women, the clear badge of sexual status has been most rigidly applied to the female sex.

In the past the most usual rule has been for unmarried girls to carry their hair loose, without ornament. Among the Franks, at the time of the Roman Empire, if a girl remained unmarried a long time, she was described as *remanet in capillo* (she remains in her hair). Married women were expected to plait their hair and adorn it with garlands, or little fillets.

The practice among Anglo-Saxons was very similar, with long, loose hair symbolizing virginity and freedom for marriage. After a certain age, even an unmarried girl might plait her hair, but on her wedding day she

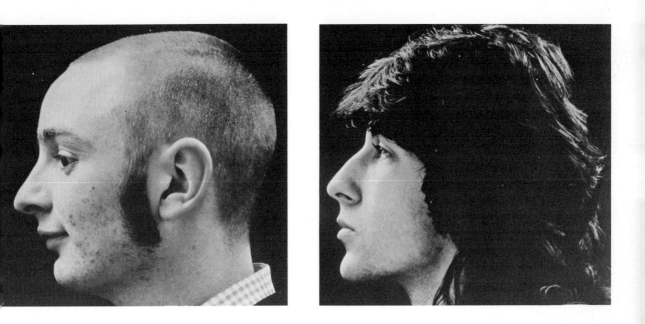

unplaited it and scattered it loose over her shoulders as the badge of her virginity. After the marriage, however, her hair had to be cut short as the badge of servitude to her husband. As civilization developed, this rather degrading practice was modified, and newly married women were required only to bind their hair in folds around the head. So loose hair continued as the mark of the unmarried woman, and bound hair of the married one, a distinction that remained in use in some rural societies until quite recent times.

In Highland Scotland, a married woman used to bind her hair with a band of white linen, and this was far more customary than a wedding ring. A widow covered her hair with a black peaked bonnet or special cap. Sir Walter Scott in his novel *The Heart of Midlothian* (1818) pointed to the problem such strict hair conventions could impose on someone outside the accepted social pattern. Writing of Effie, an unmarried mother, he referred to: "her tresses of long fair hair, which according to the costume of the country, unmarried women were not allowed to cover with any sort of cap, and which, alas! Effie dared no longer confine with the snood or ribband, which implied purity of maiden-fame . . . ."

Thus Effie had to let her hair hang completely loose and free, to distinguish her from both maid and wife. In Sweden unmarried mothers received a better deal, because according to traditional folk custom they were obliged, like married women, to cover their hair, which must have helped mask

Above left, a typical London skinhead in 1969. His head is completely cropped, except for the carefully tended sideburns. "The barber took them off once," he is reported as saying, "and I done my nut." At the same time, fashionable young men were wearing their hair romantically long (above right), thus showing in the streets of London a contrast in hair styles reminiscent of the Roundheads and Cavaliers of 300 years before.

their outcast state. Ancient Greece and Rome seemed less concerned with clearly denoting sexual status. Among the Greeks, young boys and the athletes who competed in the public games always had their hair cropped short. In full manhood the hair was worn longer, and the length and fashion of the cut served, quite as much as clothes and shoes, to indicate the polished gentleman. In general, young unmarried girls wore simpler hair styles than their mothers. In Rome, in very ancient times, the hair of newly married women was parted into six locks with a spear, and the special style later adopted by the Vestal Virgins, who tended the sacred fire at the shrine of the goddess Vesta, may have derived from this. Their hair was divided also into six parts, which were braided and wound round the head, building into a cone shape on top. In time, the strip of rough wool that had been wound around this cone of hair to symbolize the honor and dignity of the married woman gave way to linen or silk ribbons of bright colors. But the only clear distinction in Rome in later times, as we have already noted, was the compulsory fair hair which had to be worn by the prostitute as the badge of her profession.

Among Semitic people there has been a long tradition of shaving women's hair to denote the married state. The *sheitel,* as we have seen, is still worn by Orthodox Jewish women today. The custom must, in fact, be very old, for there are many references to it in Talmudic literature. Oimhith, a woman whose two sons both became high priests, accounted for this good fortune by explaining that the beams of her house had never looked upon her bare head. This custom of covering the hair or binding it close to the head to indicate a married woman probably stems from the original practice of cutting it off—in turn almost surely derived from ancient beliefs that a deity or spirit has the right to claim a maiden's virginity. The hair, loose and free, was the symbol of that virginity and had to be offered as a redemption, so that the marriage could be consummated.

Of course not all hair conventions follow this pattern. For example, unmarried girls among the hill tribes of Burma and Assam wear their hair short, and in some tribes the head is actually shaved. In contrast, married women wear their hair long. Short hair in this case may symbolize sexual restraint, in that unmarried girls are expected to avoid having children, although in these tribes premarital sexual intercourse is not only accepted but to some extent institutionalized.

It seems to have been far less common for men to bother to denote their sexual status, though the beard itself advertises sexual maturity, and facial hair is accordingly a proud badge of masculinity. Only a few cultures have used it for more precise definition. At one time it was customary in the

A contemporary cartoon guys the appearance of Existentialists in Paris in the late 1940s. The Existentialist belief that the individual is responsible only to himself, led its followers to adopt deliberately nonconformist hair styles.

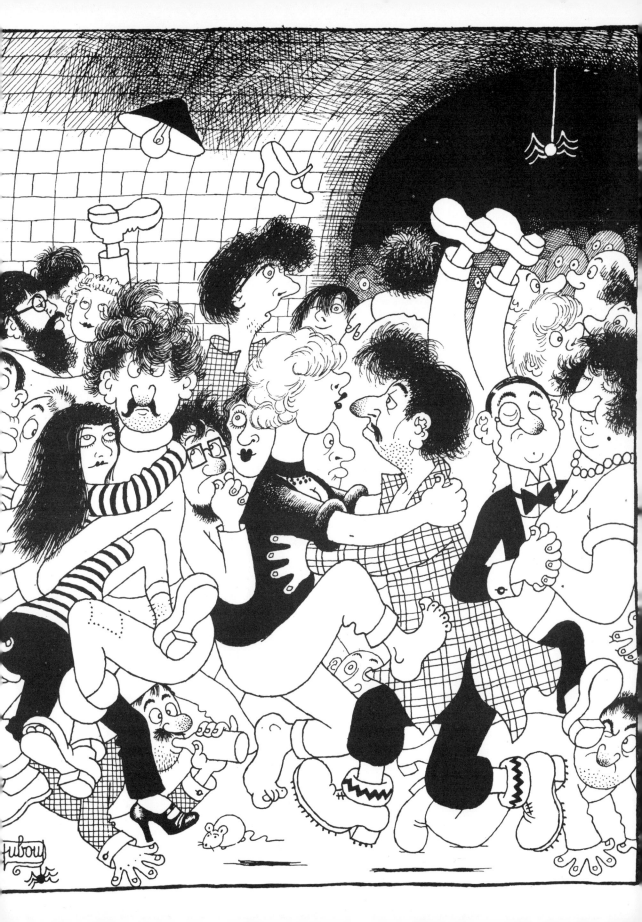

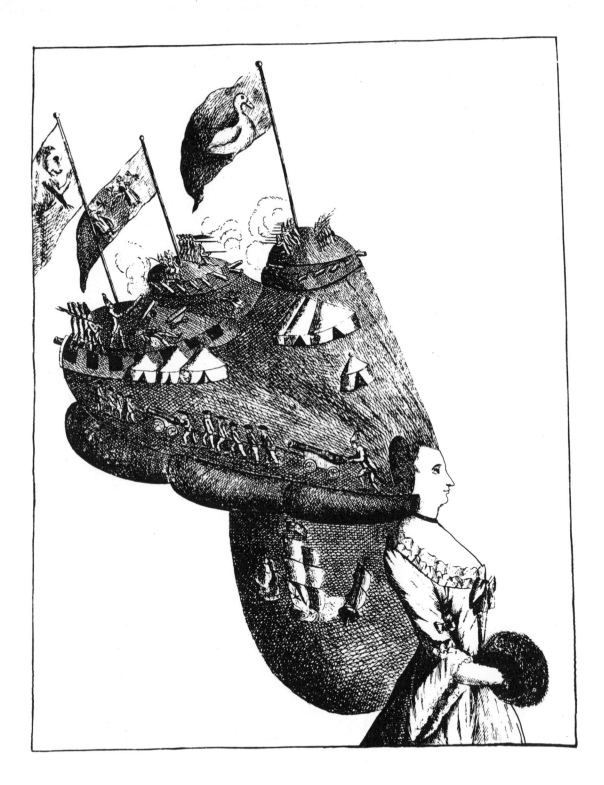

A satirical engraving of 1776 mocks the exaggerated women's hair styles that gave their wearers the opportunity to demonstrate their political (or other) loyalties. This enormous set-piece represents the defeat of the American colonists by the British forces at Bunker Hill.

Outer Hebrides, off the western coast of Scotland, for adult men to grow moustaches, but for beards to be worn only by older men who had retired from work. To this day, among the Amish sect of the Mennonites in Pennsylvania, a beard may be worn only by a married man.

It is in India among the Brahmins that hair style and sexual status in men are most closely linked, and the association is still part of contemporary culture. In an earlier chapter it has been noted that a shaven head denotes celibacy, the tonsure with a single tuft indicates sexual restraint, and the matted hair of the mystic is a badge of total sexual detachment. This symbolism is not restricted to holy men but is part of the ordinary social conventions of South Indian life.

It is extremely difficult, if not impossible, to separate the many and different functions of that most useful substance, hair. We have seen how it has been cut and shaped to indicate status, whether social, intellectual, or sexual. We have drawn attention to the tyranny of fashion, how simply to be up-to-date may provide sufficient motive for a change of style. Whatever the reason, the importance to us of the way we wear our hair has required in every age the services of experts. Today, a whole industry has developed to cater for our needs, and satisfy our fancies.

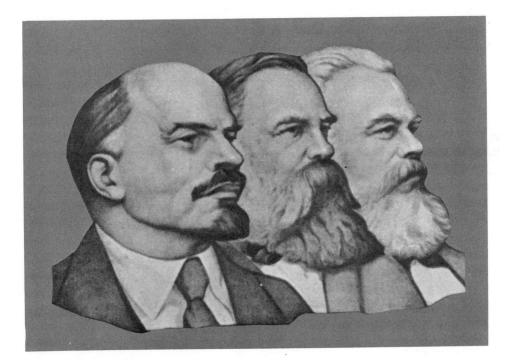

A beard is the traditional badge of the leader, the prophet, and the philosopher. Above, Nikolai Lenin (left), the revolutionary who put into practice the theories of philosopher Karl Marx (center) and his co-worker and propagandist Friedrich Engels (right).

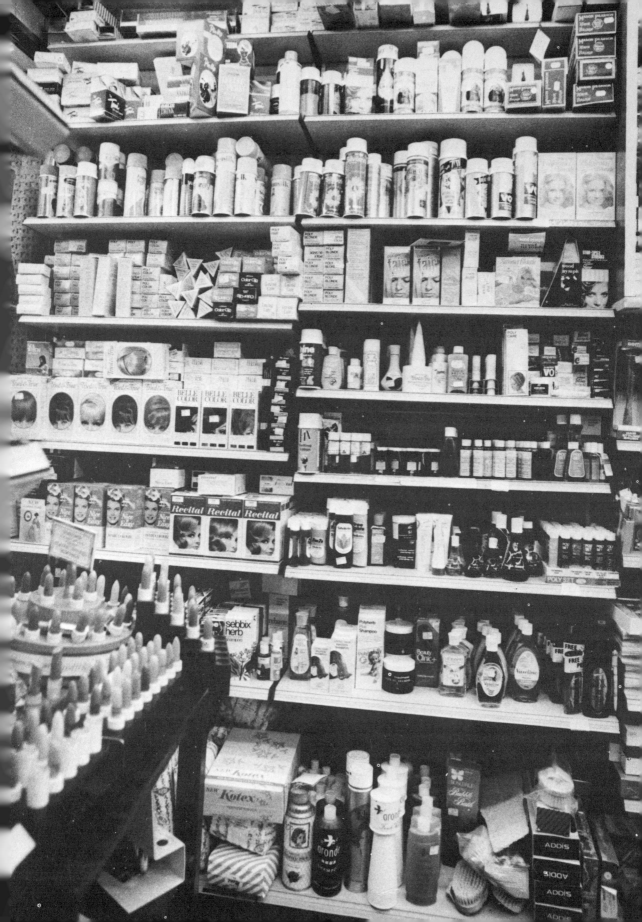

6 The Hair Industry

There is no record of how primeval man looked after his hair. Evolving from primates, he almost certainly inherited, and continued, at least for a time, their pattern of mutual grooming. We have seen that something very like this still survives among a few primitive tribes.

One thing we know, from cave paintings discovered in Mexico, is that even prehistoric men suffered from baldness. We cannot tell how widespread the problem was, nor how much it perturbed its victims. But it is clear that, certainly from the earliest historic times, baldness worried our ancestors quite as much as it does modern man. From the beginning of recorded history, there has been a continuous search for remedies, involving magic or medicine or a judicious mixture of both.

One of the earliest known cures for baldness was written down by the mother of King Chata of Egypt in about 4000 B.C. She recommended rubbing the head vigorously with a preparation made of dogs' paws, dates, and asses' hooves ground and cooked in oil. Six millennia later, with our modern knowledge of the importance of circulation to hair health, we can see that the massage may well have been beneficial, whatever the effect of the ingredients. Hippocrates himself, in about 400 B.C., offered a cure for baldness. He prescribed opium, mixed with essence of roses or lilies, and made into an ointment with wine, oil of unripe olives, or acacia juice. For more serious cases, he prescribed a poultice of cumin, pigeon droppings, crushed horseradish, and beetroot or nettles. In ancient Rome, berries of myrrh were believed to prevent baldness, and, if they failed, bears' fat was supposed to restore the hair. In the first century A.D., the physician Dioscorides wrote that to retain all one's hair it was only necessary to apply, twice a week, a concoction obtained by boiling snakes

A display of products for the hair in a London drug store. Today a multi-million-dollar industry markets hundreds of do-it-yourself products for the treatment, care, and beautification of men's and women's hair.

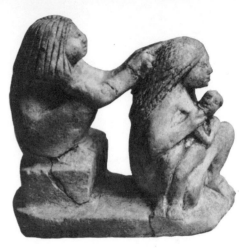

The earliest known portrayal of a hairdresser at work—an Egyptian lady nurses her baby while a slave hairdresser attends to her hair. This small limestone statuette dates from about 2000 to 1800 B.C.

alive. Vipers' oil, particularly if the snakes were caught at full moon, appears in many cultures as a hair restorer. Faced with remedies such as these, we can understand the direct approach to the problem adopted by some bald Romans, who simply painted hair on their heads with perfumed essences—"painted locks, you may shave much better with a sponge."

The ancients were anxious to discover the causes of baldness as well as its remedies. The Greek philosopher Aristotle anticipated modern knowledge of the link between baldness and the hormones by about 2000 years, although fortunately his conclusions were wrong—he thought that sexual intercourse caused baldness. Even if anyone had believed him, the implied cure would hardly have been popular. Later, in the 16th century, François Rabelais, the French priest and satirist, associated baldness with virility, and went on to anticipate modern transplant techniques by suggesting grafting as the remedy.

During the Middle Ages, monks and alchemists took up the search for a cure, and the formulae of their cosmetic secrets were jealously guarded and passed down. One Hungarian priest at the end of the 11th century used an arsenic derivative combined with a special prayer: in view of the danger of the former, the latter was a wise precaution. In the confidence and brashness of their claims the old recipes lacked nothing in comparison with modern advertising. In the ninth book of his *Natural Magick,* published in the 16th century, Giovanni Battista della Porta, under the unequivocal heading, "How Hair may grow again," quoted ancient remedies involving among other ingredients: "the Ashes of a Land Hedge hog, or of burnt Bees or Flies . . . Man's dung burnt, and anoynted with Honey." If the reader was in a special hurry to make his hair grow, della Porta recommended marsh mallow root with hog's grease, boiled in wine; and for an even quicker cure, burned barley bread, horse fat, and boiled river eel.

One renowned elixir, invented by the celebrated Swiss-born alchemist and physician Paracelsus in the 16th century, was the dark red liquid he supplied to Diane de Poitiers, mistress of Henry II of France. Although she was 50, the only sign of age that marred her beauty was thinning hair, and the mixture Paracelsus supplied to counteract this was rumored to contain blood from women in childbirth, the blood of a murdered new-born baby, and "vipers' wine."

It is small wonder that by the 17th century a young Venetian chemist, Josefo Francopolli, had the bright idea of selling dual-purpose products that were claimed, applied externally, to produce an abundant crop of hair, and, taken internally, to provide nourishment. Among his products was something called Vine Dew, enormously expensive, and discovered to consist mostly of water from the river Seine. Discredited and banished from the court of Versailles, Francopolli moved to the court of the King of Naples, where, quite undiscouraged, he launched a new product, Calf Water, to cure falling hair, and pursued his secondary career of seduction. At the age of 74, still going strong in both arts, he was killed in a duel, just as his latest hair speciality, Octopus Fat, was gaining popularity.

Many of the potions and lotions used on the scalp must have had disastrous results. This was particularly true of fast-acting dyes. Ovid unsympathetically reproached one Roman lady who had ruined her hair in this way. He wrote: "Your own hand has been the cause of the loss you deplore. You poured the poison on your own head. Now Germany will send you slaves' hair. A vanquished nation will supply your ornament."

Despite Ovid's words, it was probably not the lady's own hand that did the pouring. The vanquished nations supplied more than ornaments; they supplied slaves. Throughout ancient Egypt, Greece, and Rome, household slaves dressed their masters' and mistresses' hair and shaved their masters. Men who did not possess slaves, or who preferred to gossip to friends while being shaved, could use itinerant barbers or barbers' shops.

Hairdressing has a long history. It is frequently mentioned in the literature and depicted in the paintings of many ancient cultures. One biblical reference comes in Ezekiel V:1: "And thou, son of man, take thee a sharp knife, take thee a barber's razor, and cause it to pass upon thine head and upon thy beard." Perhaps the most surprising aspect of ancient hairdressing is how sophisticated it was. Ancient shaving sets have been found in Egypt, dating from 2000 B.C. or earlier, containing bronze razors, tweezers, and hair curlers, hones made of grit stone, bronze mirrors with ivory handles, shaving mugs, combs, and hairpins. It is suspected that the Egyptians must have had a method of tempering copper and bronze to achieve a really good cutting edge, although, if so, the knowledge was subsequently lost. They were certainly tremendous shavers, for shaven heads were practically universal among men, and priests and high officials shaved the entire body. Wigs were widely worn by both sexes, the best made of human hair, but others often of wool, cotton, or palm-leaf fibers. Many were dyed with henna or indigo. They were often braided, and set with beeswax—at dinner parties, cakes of perfumed wax were placed on the wigs of guests. The melting wax was supposed to provide a cooling effect. The street barber was common in Egypt; his customers would kneel at the side of the road while he shaved their heads.

The ancient Greeks were well versed in the art of hairdressing. When Alexander the Great forbade his soldiers to wear beards in 323 B.C., the clean-shaven fashion spread to the civilian population, and barbers' shops, which were open to the street, flourished; but ladies' hair continued to be tended by slaves. Barbers not only cut and curled head hair, but removed body hair, which was very much disliked. The Greek historian Theopompos, in the 4th century B.C., described how "among the Tyrrhenians [Etruscans] there are many shops for this purpose and well-trained staffs, as in our barbers' shops. Persons enter these shops and let themselves be treated in any way on any part of the body without troubling about the looks of passers-by." It all sounds very sociable and informal, and we know that Greek barbers' shops were often well-appointed and even luxurious places. After his early morning bath, the Greek townsman would stroll to his barber as part of his social round and meet friends and travelers from abroad, exchange news, and discuss politics.

In Rome the upper classes were mostly shaved by their slaves, but the rest of the men, like the Greeks, went to public barbers' shops. With slaves as cheap assistants, barbers could make a great deal of money. Juvenal speaks of one who owned innumerable villas, and Martial mentions another whose wife achieved rapid promotion for him by means of the large bribes he was able to pay out. According to the historian Livy, the first Roman to shave was the legendary King Tarquin the Elder, in the sixth century B.C. But the fashion for clean-shaven chins took hold only in 297 B.C., after the arrival in Rome of a troop of barbers from Sicily— although the general Scipio Africanus (237–183 B.C.) is reputed to have been the first Roman to shave daily.

Blond hair was fashionable in Rome for long periods. Ovid describes how the desired fairness was achieved by the use of "German herbs." The elder Pliny left a much more unpleasant formula for black hair dye, made up of leeches and vinegar fermented together for two months in a lead

Right, a street barber at work in India. Street barbers were common in ancient Egypt, but—once the Romans had demonstrated the greater comfort of covered barber's shops—they seem never to have established themselves in Europe. They still exist, however, in many parts of the East.

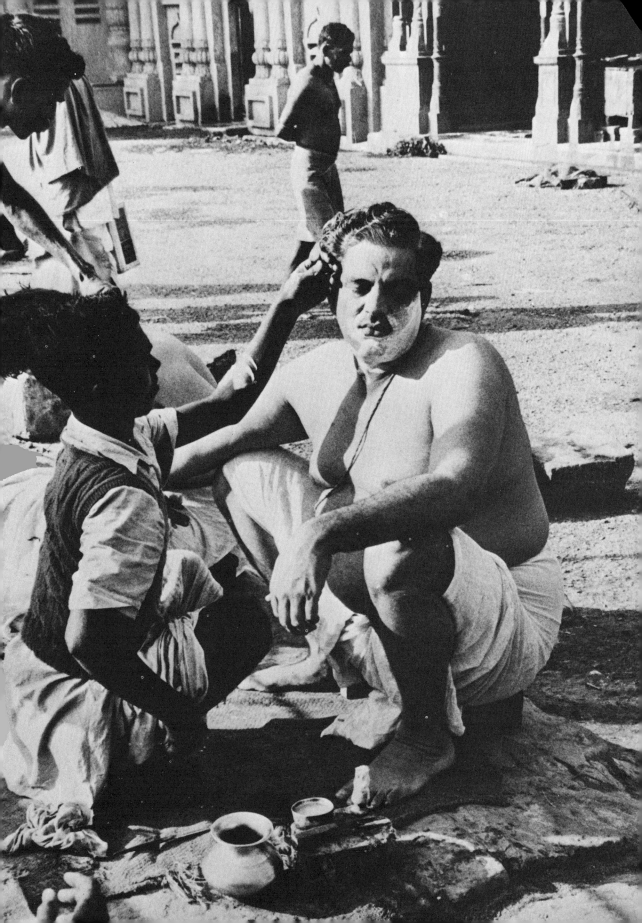

vessel. Roman hairdressers understood the art of tinting and bleaching, and they also discovered warm-water shaving. They used flat, straight razors, and treated the beard with an oily preshave lotion. It sounds quite contemporary, until we remember that a favorite pastime of the second-century Emperor Commodus was to commandeer a barber's shop and amuse himself by cutting off the customers' noses.

Women's hair was elaborately dressed by specialist slaves, each with his own descriptive title. The slaves who used the *calamistrum,* or curling iron, for example, were known as *ciniflones*. Splendid effects were achieved with these irons, and with wigs, false hair, braids, and nets, all secured by single-pronged hairpins of gold, silver, jet, bone, or ivory, topped with jeweled or carved heads.

After the collapse of the Roman Empire in the West during the fifth century A.D., there are few records concerning the history of hairdressing until the early 14th century. During the early part of this period—generally termed the Dark Ages—it seems likely that the barber's shop, which was a familiar institution in ancient Rome, disappeared. But within the monasteries, the old cosmetic secrets and cures were preserved, spiced (as we have seen) with religious superstition. But by the 11th century the barber had come back into his own. In 1092 a papal decree required the clergy to be clean-shaven, and the barber became a familiar figure in the

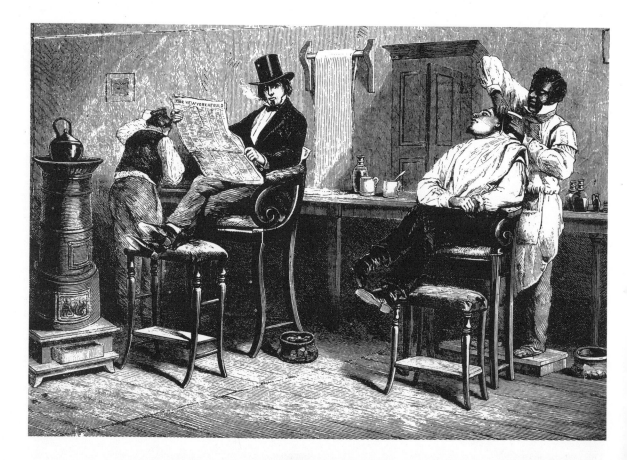

monasteries. During the Dark Ages, monks had practiced medicine and surgery, but in 1163 the Council of Tours banned the shedding of blood by the clergy, and the barbers, because of their skill with the razor, were their natural successors. In England, London barbers displayed jars of blood in their windows to advertise this section of their trade, but in 1307 this practice was forbidden—henceforth the blood had to be deposited in the river Thames.

The first public register of barber-surgeons was drawn up in France in 1301, when 26 of them banded together. Shortly afterwards, in 1308, Richard le Barbour was sworn in as the first Master of the Barbers Company of England. The company increased in importance and in 1462, the first year of Edward IV's reign, barbers were incorporated by royal charter. In 1540, during the reign of Henry VIII, surgeons and barbers were jointly incorporated as the Barber-Surgeons Company.

For many centuries there was great rivalry between the surgeons and the barbers. In France during the 14th century, physicians refused to admit barbers to the Faculty of Medicine. Together with the surgeons, they unsuccessfully attempted to monopolize all rights of tending the sick. In England an enactment in the reign of Henry VIII stated that "no person using any shaving or barbery in London shall occupy any surgery, letting of blood, or other matter, except drawing of teeth." Similarly, the surgeons were barred from "barbery or shaving." The enactment was to no avail, for both sides continued to encroach on each other's territory. The two functions were finally separated by Act of Parliament in 1745, although even then a few barber-surgeons lingered on, the last one—reputedly named Middleditch—dying in 1821.

The rivalry between the doctors and barbers was to cast a long shadow, for it meant that few doctors would demean themselves to bother with what they considered the low-grade problems of hair and scalp. As medicine began to progress from an art to something approaching a science, the care of hair was left in the hands of charlatans, and treatments involved a mumbo jumbo of alchemy, magic, and superstition.

By the 16th century, men's barbers' shops had come to resemble those of classical times. We have seen that the Greeks and Romans enjoyed the social atmosphere of the barber's, and the same is true of Elizabethan England. Young gallants came in not just to have their beards trimmed and perhaps their sword wounds dressed, but to get the latest news and even to enjoy music. A cittern or guitar would be on the counter, and customers played and sang while awaiting their turn. According to one contemporary account, a barber is "all the while keeping time on his

A New York barber's shop in the late 19th century—a place to talk, meet friends, and catch up with the news as well as to be shaved and have the beard and hair trimmed.

cittern; for you know a cittern to a barber is as natural as milk to a calf, or bears to be attended by bagpipes." The barber was often a man of considerable intelligence and local importance. He not only cut hair, trimmed wigs, bled the sick, pulled teeth, and dressed wounds, but, in an age when there was no mass distribution of newspapers, passed on to his customers news of local events and scandals.

Robert Greene, the 16th-century English poet and dramatist, gives a vivid picture of the ceremonial of the barber's shop in his *Quip for an Upstart Courtier,* published in 1592. He relates how the barber greets his courtier customer with a bow, and asks: "Sir, will you have your worship's hair cut after the Italian manner, shorte and round, and then frounst with the curling yrons, to make it looke like a halfe moone in a mist; or like a Spanyard, long at the eares, and curled like to the two endes of an olde cast periwig; or will you be Frenchefied with a love locke downe to your shoulders, wherein you may weare your mistresse's favour? The English cut is base, and gentlemen scorne it; novelty is daintye. Speake the word, sir, my sissars are ready to execute your worship's will."

A couple of hours were spent combing and dressing the hair, and then the barber's basin was washed with camphor soap, and the bowing and inquiring began again. According to Greene, the barber "descends as low as his beard, and asketh whether he please to be shaven or no; whether he will have his peak cut shorte and sharpe, amiable like an inamorato or broade pendant like a spade, to be terrible like a warrior and a soldado; whether he will have his crates cut lowe like a Juniper bush, or his suberches taken away with a razor; if it be his pleasure to have his appendices primde, or his moustachaces fostered to turn about his eares like the branches of a vine, or cut downe to the lip with the Italian lashe?" And with every question a snip of the scissors and a bow. But if a poor man entered the shop, he would be unceremoniously "polled for twopence," and trimmed around "like the halfe of a Holland cheese."

Like all good clubs the barbers' shops had rules, which were conspicuously displayed, and penalties for breaking them. Forfeits had to be paid for handling razors, talking of cutting throats, calling hair powder flour, or meddling with anything on the barber's work board. That no one took the rules very seriously is suggested by Shakespeare's simile in *Measure for Measure:*

> . . . like the forfeits in a barber's shop,
> As much in mock as mark.

Perhaps the best-known of all barbers is the legendary Sweeney Todd of Fleet Street in London. First heard of in the 19th century and perpetuated

An advertisement of the early 1900s for a popular British hair tonic.

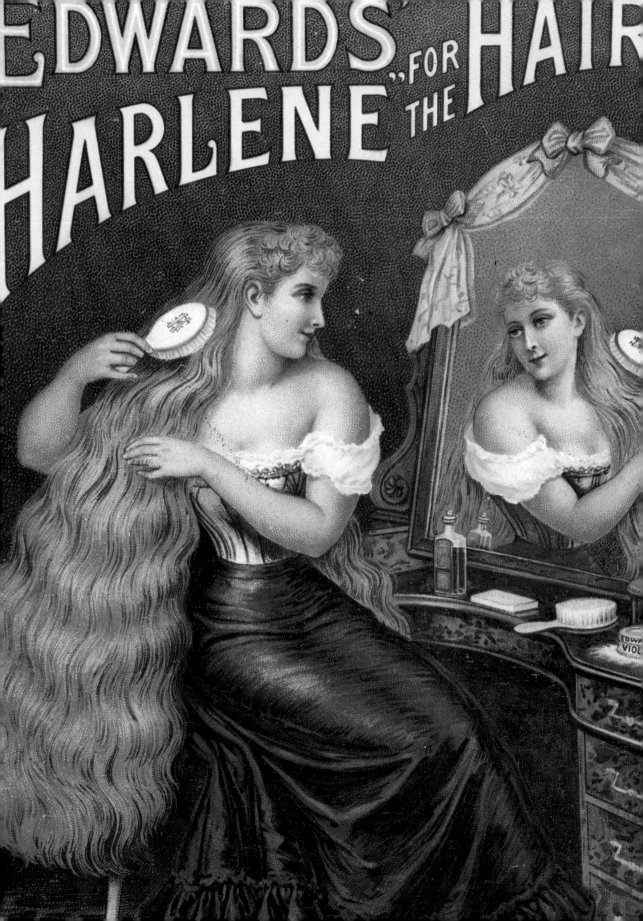

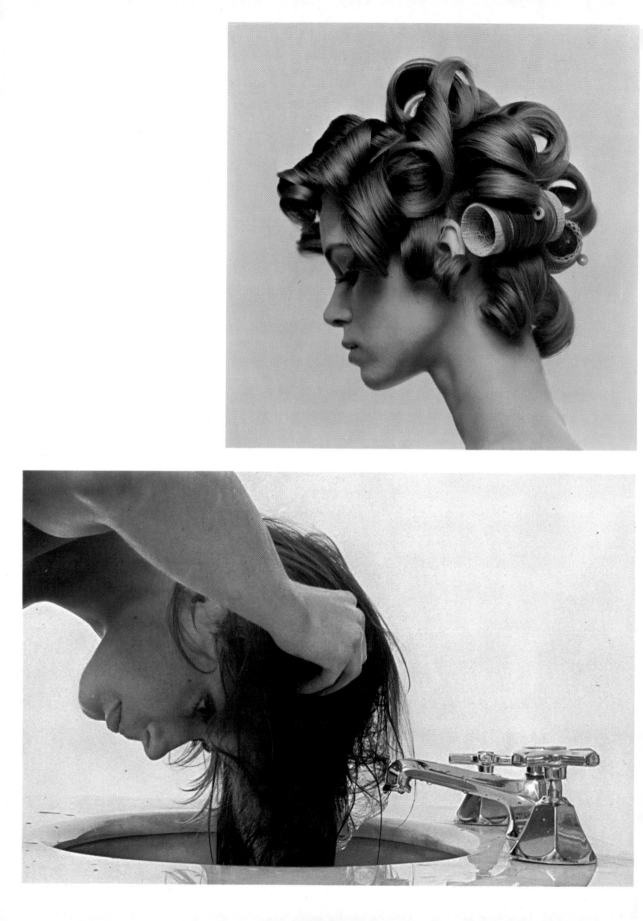

in popular melodrama as "the demon barber," he was what we should now call an anti-hero, and no credit to his trade. According to the original story, one barber's chair in his shop stood on a trapdoor in the floor. If a customer came in who seemed worth robbing, Sweeney would show him to this chair. "Then suddenly the chair would turn a half somersault, hurling the occupant into a cellar fifteen feet deep, and paved with sharp edges of stone placed in a perpendicular position." If the fall failed to kill, Sweeney would slit his victim's throat with a razor. Sweeney Todd's French counterpart was a notorious *assassin-perruquier* of Paris. This gentleman, after dispatching his victims, disposed of their bodies to his next-door neighbor, a pastry-cook, whose shop in the rue de la Harpe became famous for its savory patties.

Another Parisian barber, Joseph Orcher, whose job it was to attend daily at the residence of the Marquis de Courzi, slit this noble's throat, and escaped to Martinique in the West Indies with 100 gold louis. Under the name of Lestange he married a titled heiress, but made the mistake 29 years later of returning to Paris, believing that by then he would not be recognized. He was, and ended his life on the guillotine. If he had stayed away just 8 months longer, to complete the 30 years prescribed by the statute of limitation, he would have been safe from indictment.

Women barbers, who are today coming back into fashion, were by no means unknown in the past. An English writer, William Andrews, in his book *At the Sign of the Barber's Pole* (1904), mentions five women barbers who lived in Drury Lane in London at the time of Charles II. The 17th-century English biographer John Aubrey tells a story about one of these women, who infected a neighbor's husband with the pox. The wife was rightly outraged. She and her neighbors decided to punish the guilty barber and "concluded on this Revenge, viz. to gett her and whippe her and to shave all the haire off her pudenda; which severities were executed." The episode inspired a popular ballad, whose chorus ran:

> Did yee ever heare the like
> Or ever heard the same
> Of five Woemen-Barbers
> That lived in Drewry-lane?

At the beginning of the 19th century a street near the Strand was the haunt of "black women," reputed to shave "with ease and dexterity," while St. Giles'-in-the-Fields also boasted a female shaver. J. T. Smith mentions in his *Ancient Topography of London* (1815) being shaved by a woman "at the Seven Dials in Great St. Andrew's Street," while her husband, a strapping soldier in the Horse Guards, sat smoking his pipe.

By the late 1950s more and more women were dressing their hair at home rather than attending a professional hairdresser. Hair rollers (top) allowed the unskilled to set their own curls and waves and a variety of shampoos for all types of hair made hair-washing (bottom) easy.

Although the trimming of beards and moustaches, when they were in fashion, was largely carried out by barbers, the really wealthy relied upon their personal servants. Mrs. Beeton, who wrote the famous 19th-century cookery book, also listed the essential qualifications for a valet to a gentleman of the period: "He should be a good hairdresser. He has to brush the hair, beard and moustaches, arranging the whole simply and gracefully according to the style preferred."

The powdering of hair and wigs was something that called for great ingenuity, particularly where the natural hair was blended in with a wig. The powder was blown on with bellows by a valet or wig-maker, while a cape or apron was worn, and the face buried in a cone or protected by a mask. All well-do-do houses had powder closets where this rather messy operation could be performed.

Wig-making, of course, was at times an important part of the barber's trade, and never more so than in the 17th and 18th centuries. It was such a flourishing business that in France in 1665 its practitioners became established in a separate guild from the barber-surgeons. We have seen that, at first, wigs were elaborate and expensive, and only the wealthy and fashionable could afford them. After a time, a fashion for smaller wigs spread, and they came within the means of the middle and even lower classes. By the mid-18th century a common wig could be purchased for less than a guinea, and even an ordinary journeyman treated himself to a new one every year. Apprentice indentures usually contained a clause ensuring that the master should provide "one good and sufficient wig yearly during the term of apprenticeship."

The better wigs were made of human hair, most of it imported. The diarist Samuel Pepys, on 18 July 1664, records rebuking his barber for delivering him a wig that was full of nits. The Great Plague of 1665 brought worse dangers, and Pepys noted: "Up and put on my coloured silk suit, very fine, and my new periwigg, bought a good while since, but durst not wear, because the plague was in Westminster when I bought it; and it is a wonder what will be the fashion, after the plague is done, as to periwiggs, for nobody will dare to buy any hayre for fear of the infection, that it had been cut off the heads of people dead of the plague."

Both Pepys and the periwigs survived the plague, and with the fashion spreading to America, wig-makers were busier than ever supplying made-to-measure wigs for the owners of large American estates. Eventually, to supply the less wealthy, a local industry became established and many London craftsmen emigrated to the colonies. In Williamsburg, the capital of Virginia, at least eight wig-makers were at work in 1769.

Right, a micro-skirted girl hairdresser at work in a barber's shop in 1970. Women barbers are not a product of 20th-century permissiveness. Far right, women hairdressers in an English barber's shop in about 1700. Their client's head has been covered with a cap while his wig is being combed.

Cheaper wigs were sometimes made of animal hair, and occasionally even of feathers. One peruke-maker's advertisement read: "Very durable wigs, not to be hurt at least by wet, made of the single feathers in mallard's tails." Another enterprising peruke-maker was reported in an English newspaper, the *Ipswich Journal*, in May 1750, as having invented "a wig of copper wire which will resist all weathers and last for ever."

But the fashion for wigs was *not* to last for ever. Their use had become too widespread and toward the end of the 18th century the elite was experimenting again with that amazing discovery, natural hair. As the wig-makers saw the first sign of this affecting their trade, they set up a wail of protest. In 1765 they anticipated modern methods and staged a protest march. They petitioned the king, George III, to enforce the wearing of wigs by law. As a number of them wore no wig themselves, they were hardly setting much of an example, and the London crowd became so irritated that they "seized the petitioners, and cut off all their hair per force." Even worse for the poor wig-makers was the ridicule heaped on them by wags of the period, who suggested that carpenters should protest against the lack of demand for wooden legs. They even published a petition, purporting to come from the carpenters, begging His Majesty to wear a wooden leg, and urging his courtiers to follow suit.

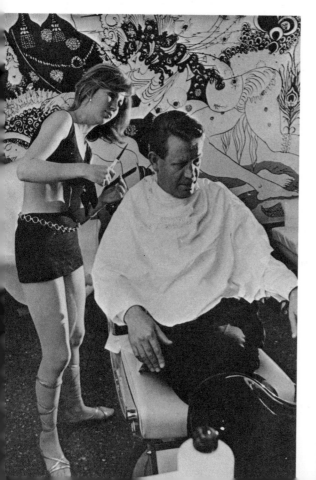

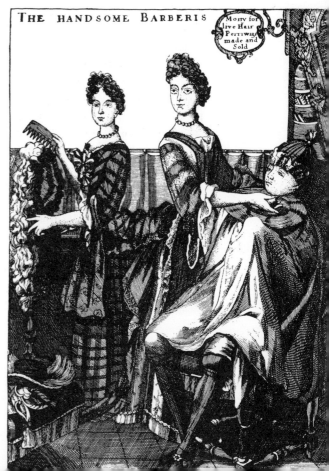

Whereas barbers' shops have been a male institution since classical times, no equivalent seems to have existed for women until the present century. However, there emerged in 17th century France a line of great artist-hairdressers—a line that continues to this day.

The first—or the first whose name is known to us—was Champagne. Born in the south of France, of humble parents, he is supposed to have begun his career as a boy by arranging the hair of a young shepherdess who had injured her right arm on a scythe. The hair style caught the eye of a countess, who took the boy into her service, and later to Paris. Once there, Champagne clearly sensed his destiny, for to everyone's surprise he opened a salon for ladies' hair. Until then only women's hands had dressed women's hair, and the Church at once censured this new departure as highly immoral. Then, as now, this sort of condemnation proved to be valuable publicity, and the idea caught on. Although Champagne never took money, he did extremely well out of lavish gifts, including a coach from ex-Queen Christina of Sweden.

Because Champagne is credited with founding the profession of ladies' coiffeur, and because many of today's temperamental and independent top hairdressers still seem to be cast in his image, it is worth recording the contemporary picture of him given by the writer Tallemant des Reaux. He wrote: "This prig Champagne, by his cleverness in dressing the hair, and by his pushing ways, was run after and caressed by all the ladies. Their weakness for him rendered him so important as to address to them a hundred insolences every day. Some he left with their hair half dressed; with others he dressed their hair on one side, and then demanded a kiss before he would do the other side. Sometimes he would leave, saying he should not return unless some person who had displeased him, were sent away, as he could not achieve anything artistic while she was looking on . . . . When dressing a lady, he would mention what so-and-so had given him, and when he had not been satisfied he would add: 'She may send for me again, but I don't intend to go.' The poor lady who heard it would tremble with fear, lest he should desert her also, and she would give him double what she had intended to."

Champagne died in 1658 (killed by brigands on his way to the south of France) and had no immediate successor. A little later in the century, a Madame Martin emerged as the rage in Paris, and began to build up women's hair high instead of wide, the previous fashion. But it was a former cook turned hairdresser, Legros de Rumigny, who, in the next century, really transformed an art into a profession. He published in 1766 a book so successful that it ran into four editions, and no woman of

Right, a late 18th-century caricature of an English gentleman protecting his face with a paper cone while his valet powders his wig. Far right, a 16th-century woodcut shows shampooing and haircutting in a barber's shop of the period.

fashion dared to try to live without it. He founded an *Académie de Coiffure,* which ran classes for prospective coiffeurs and coiffeuses, who paid six louis, and were taught 38 of Legros' original designs. Classes for valets involved 28 designs and four louis, while the lowest class for mere chambermaids cost only two louis, but omitted any instruction on hair-cutting. His pupils practiced Legros' styles on the hair of pretty girls called *prêteuses de têtes* (head lenders), who were expected on public occasions to display both his new creations and the skill of his pupils.

Despite all this business-like professionalism, superstition still confused logic, for Legros recommended that in order to preserve the natural hair, the ends should be cut at every new moon, though not at the red moon. Hairdressers of the time no doubt lived well, but they seem to have died violently; poor Legros was crushed to death accidentally during celebrations in honor of the marriage of the future Louis XVI to Marie Antoinette. His death may have saved him from professional eclipse, for a rival, Frédéric, was on the way up. At court other names topped the bill. Marie Antoinette appointed Larseneur as her hairdresser, but found he did not satisfy her taste, and it throws a kindly light on a queen often deemed vain and heartless to know that rather than dismiss the aging Larseneur, who relied on her patronage for his living, she allowed him to continue dressing her hair, bringing in her new favorite Léonard to completely redo it in secret afterwards. When Larseneur retired, Léonard took over and the queen gave him permission to dress the hair of other

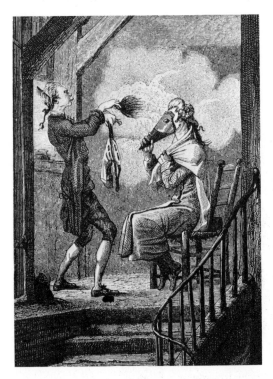

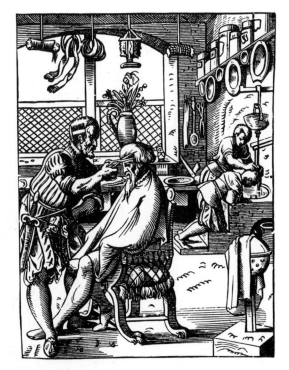

ladies—a thing that had never been allowed before. It is said that Léonard rather cleverly convinced the queen that his fingers would lose their dexterity unless he was able to practice on others.

So much was Léonard in the confidence of Marie Antoinette that in 1791 he was one of those charged with preparing the relays of horses, and forwarding a case of jewelry to Brussels, for the unsuccessful flight of the royal family that ended in capture at Varennes. Perhaps he was a better coiffeur than conspirator, for although the jewels arrived, the relays of horses failed, and with them the hopes of the royal family. Léonard himself evaded the pursuit of the revolutionaries and reached Russia, where he proved as successful as he had been in Paris.

Even before the French Revolution, women of the wealthy bourgeois class had imitated court fashions and had employed the same hairdressers. They looked to the Revolution to stamp out the aristocratic class that outshone them, but they had no desire to stamp out aristocratic fashions and luxuries. They simply took them over. Throughout the 18th century, France dictated fashion not only in Europe but in America as well. Everything *à la mode* was by definition *à la Parisienne*. The new imperial nobility of Napoleon maintained the high standards. In 1804, the German dramatist von Kotzebue declared in his *Souvenirs de Paris:* "A Parisienne requires 365 coiffures, as many pairs of shoes, six hundred dresses, and twelve chemises." She also required the services of the artist-hairdresser, who continued to be a power in the land, and still drove around to the great house in his private coach. The *Journal de Paris* of October 1805

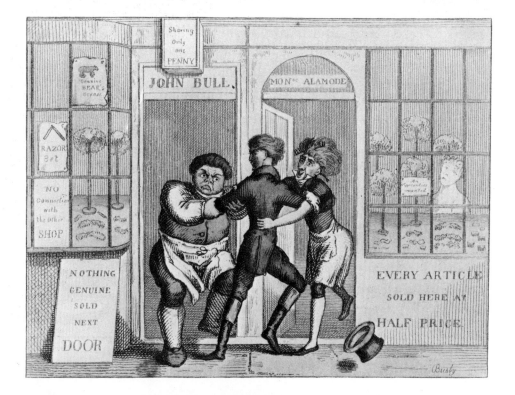

reported: "These artist-hairdressers are becoming of more importance every day. Since ladies have discontinued the use of powder the coiffure has become more difficult to arrange."

In the 20th century they are still important. The great procession of artist-hairdressers that Champagne began still clips and curls away at the heads of the world's female elite—Alexandre and Carita in Paris, Sergio and Alba and Francesca in Rome, Kenneth in New York, Masters in Beverley Hills, René, Sassoon, and Leonard in London, Möller in Hamburg. They still wait upon the thinning ranks of the very rich and the very royal in their homes and palaces, or, like Britain's Vidal Sassoon, fly 6000 miles to Hollywood to cut a super-star's hair for a single film. But all the same a quiet revolution has taken place in the 20th century. With the advent of the ladies' hairdressing salon, the clients, even quite important ones, now wait upon the hairdresser.

Looking back, it seems strange that although barbers' shops have been numerous in every age, there has never been any equivalent for women until recent times. Only with the growing emancipation of women early in this century did ladies' hairdressing salons begin to appear. At first they operated mainly in capital cities and bigger towns, but eventually they proliferated in every suburb and village, often boasting, with little or no justification, the name of some top hairdresser of the day.

But this massive expansion and democratization of a once exclusive profession has not disturbed the artist-hairdresser from his pinnacle of talent and success. He is still patronized by the famous and the rich, and he is now able to set styles for the masses. His curls and swirls, his fads and fringes, his cuts and lops, all his wild creative inspirations, are envied and copied by aspiring and perspiring assistants in salons throughout the world. In Paris, Alexandre has continued in the grand tradition, dedicated to his art and to his exclusive clientele, which includes Princess Grace of Monaco, the Duchess of Windsor, Juliette Greco, Claudia Cardinale, and a hundred glamorous names from the world of celebrities. He leaves us in no doubt about his creed when he declares: "The base of the art of the coiffure is the cut, as the foundation of a building is the base of architecture . . . . A woman in our times is ugly only if she chooses to be. Any un-attractive feature can be disguised by a good hair style." And the new hair styles he creates are displayed almost exactly as were those of Legros 200 years ago, first by top mannequins, and then by 10 of his favorite clients whom Alexandre asks to appear at a soirée. If they report the new coiffures a success, which according to Alexandre they do 95 per cent of the time, a new fashion is launched.

Keen competition between two London barbers—an 18th-century engraving.

In New York, the newly appointed French director of the Caruso salon displayed all the independence of the redoubtable Champagne when he insisted: "I want to *create* coiffures for a woman, not to have her tell me what she wants." And yet, in some mysterious way, the old tradition of confidence is maintained. A woman still thinks of her hairdresser as a trusted friend, and will let her hair down in his salon in more ways than one. She may not literally put her life into his hands as Marie Antoinette did, but she may entrust to him her happiness and her reputation.

We must not allow the maintenance of the tradition of trust between hairdresser and client to obscure the fact that today certain aspects of the hair industry are really big business—for instance, wig-making. We left the wig-makers in 1765 protesting at what they foresaw was the decline of the wig fashion. Only recently has the industry burgeoned once again, although this time its customers are mostly women. Modern wig manufacture is centered not in Paris or London, but chiefly in Hong Kong. Both economics and experience have dictated the location, for ancient Chinese skills, low wages, new Japanese machinery, and a plentiful supply of long hair from the east, have combined to make Hong Kong the wig capital of the world. In 1969 there were over 300 factories on the island, exporting more than $100 million worth of wigs, and that figure was more than 100 per cent up on the previous year.

In 1968 sales of wigs in the USA, from all sources, were estimated at 500 million dollars. The introduction of synthetic hair in the late 1950s brought prices tumbling down and greatly expanded demand. Hundreds of companies sprang up in the USA to manufacture, import, and distribute wigs. One big company, Fashion Tress, sold nearly 6 million dollars' worth of wigs in 1968, and expected sales to reach 11 million dollars in 1970.

Although some wigs cost 200 to 300 dollars, and sometimes even 1000 dollars, the trend is toward wigs and hairpieces so inexpensive that they can be considered dispensable, encouraging continuous replacement sales. Although the best and most expensive wigs are still made by hand and use human hair, the medium price range is "wefted," a machine process with a hand finish. The cheaper wigs are made of acrylic fiber, which is sent out to Hong Kong to be made up. The 107 standard shades for wigs were originally established in France and range from jet black at number 1 to pale silver gray at number 107.

Raw hair used in the wig industry comes chiefly from mainland China, India, and Indonesia. In fact, wherever people are poor, hair is for sale. In India, where pilgrims offer their hair at the temple of Venkateswara, 1000 miles southeast of New Delhi, priests sell it to a government-controlled

Opposite: some of the Western-style hair styles offered to men in the breakaway state of Biafra in 1969, during the Nigerian civil war. Overleaf, styles for women in the same village barber's shop.

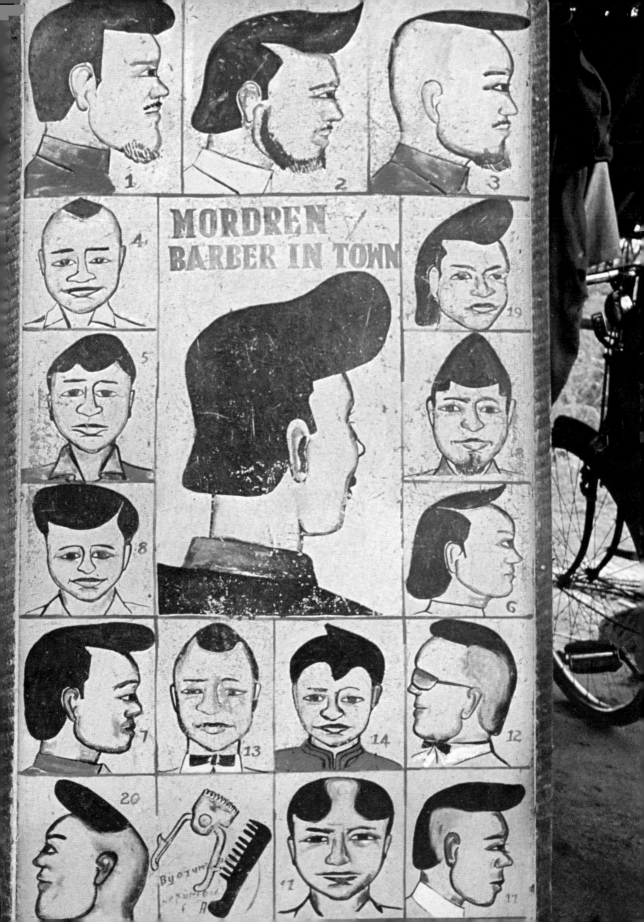

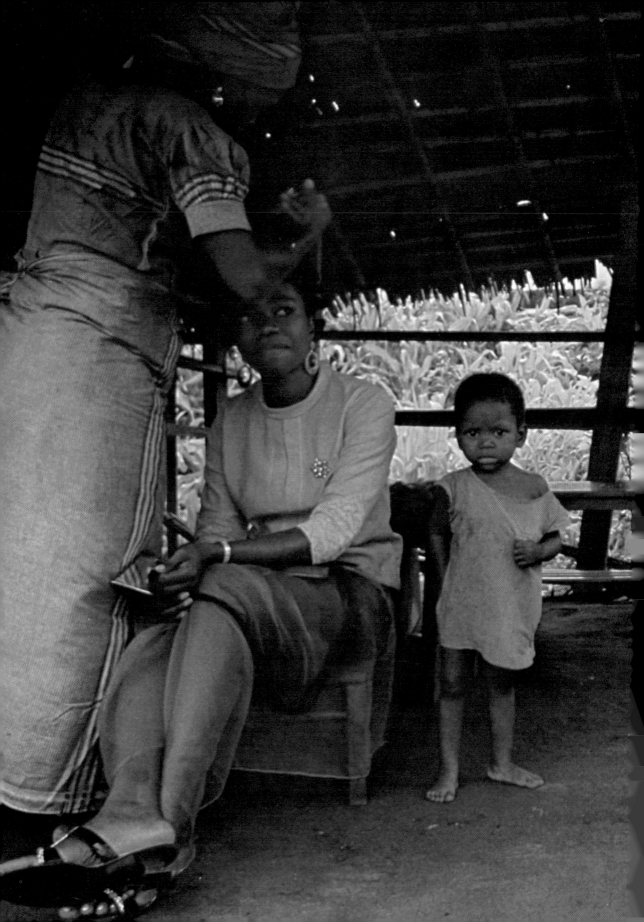

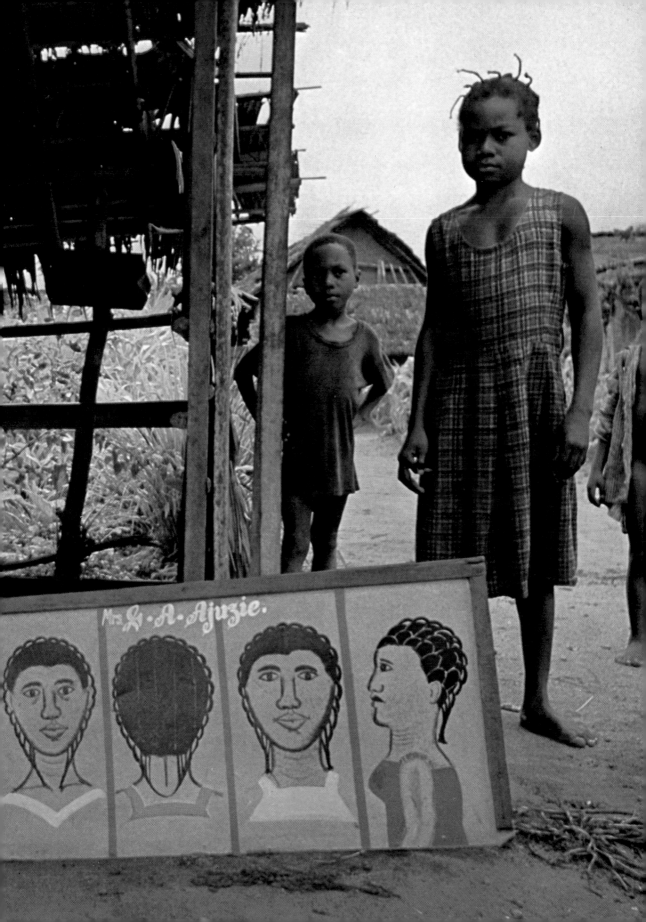

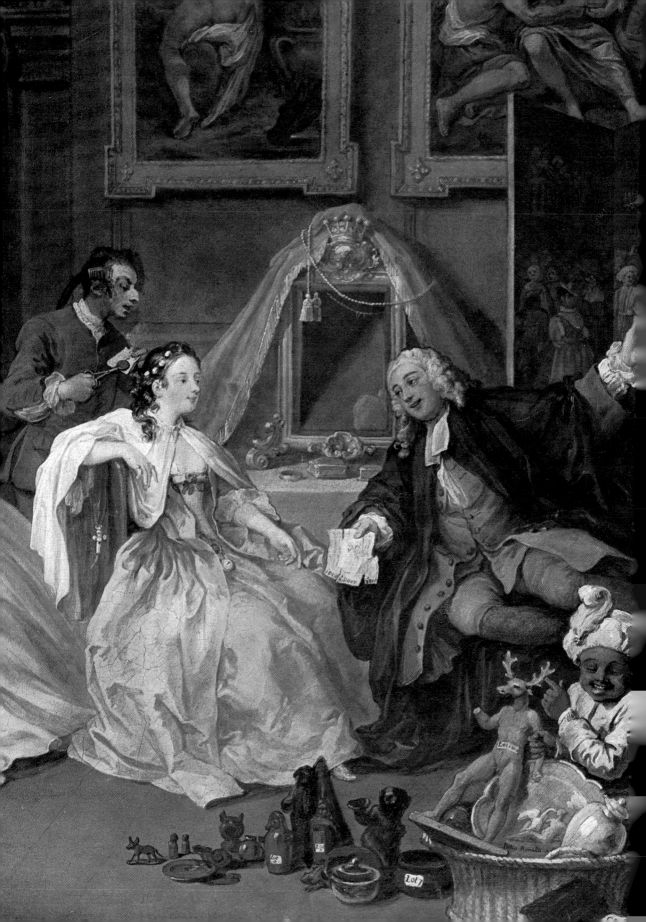

industry that makes it into wigs for export to the USA. But today more and more wigs are being made from synthetic hair. In 1968 Hong Kong manufacturers exported to the USA 38 million dollars' worth of wigs made from human hair. In 1969, of total exports of wigs amounting to 65 million dollars, nearly half were of synthetic hair.

In America it was estimated in 1968 that 75 to 80 per cent of women in the large cities and affluent suburbs owned hairpieces of one kind or another. In Great Britain in 1969 over the country as a whole, 13 per cent of all women owned a wig. It has become clear that the 16- to 24-year-olds, who are somewhat resistant to regular professional hairdressing, are finding a solution in inexpensive synthetic wigs. Real hair wigs need skilled attention at the hairdressers, but the acrylic ones are waterproof, and hold their set permanently. British imports from Hong Kong of wigs in 1969 added up to £8 million (22.5 million dollars), and the figure is still rising. Wigs can be bought in England for as little as £3 (7 dollars) in big stores, or in the wig boutiques that have mushroomed throughout the country.

But the new target for the wig-maker is the male. In America a manufacturer recently estimated that some 20 per cent of bald-headed men are wearing toupees. In Britain also there is a brisk trade, and the 40,000 men who wear hairpieces are not all actors or public figures. Knotted into a silk or nylon base, or tufted into fiber glass, men's wigs are accurately made to cover the balding area and to match surrounding hair. Attached with adhesive, they stand up to reasonable wear and tear, but are normally removed for sleeping, and must not be allowed to get wet.

Although the made-to-measure toupee is expensive, often costing from 100 to 400 dollars, the ready-to-wear or synthetic hairpieces are much cheaper, but do not blend so naturally. In any case, costly or cheap, they still have to be removed at night, and the owner is never able to forget the bald head beneath. The real psychological breakthrough has come with an entirely new process called hairweaving. This involves attaching extra hairs to those that still remain. It was originated by a black hairdresser in New York, who grew tired of straightening her clients' Negro hair, and cut it off instead, weaving straight European hair into the remaining short lengths. Hair added in this way can be washed, combed, smoothed by hand, immersed in a swimming pool or the sea, and generally treated like natural hair, without fear of it shrinking or shifting. Best of all, the bald head beneath need never be seen again. The one snag is that six times a year it must be "regroomed." Because the woven additional hairs are attached to growing hairs, they have to be periodically unlinked and reattached further down. The original weaving takes some four hours,

A detail from one of the paintings in the series Marriage à la Mode *by William Hogarth (1697-1764). A foppish ladies' hairdresser curls his client's hair during her morning toilet—carried out in a room crowded with visitors.*

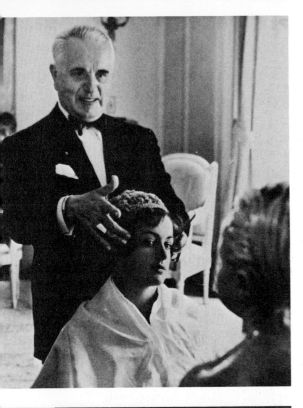

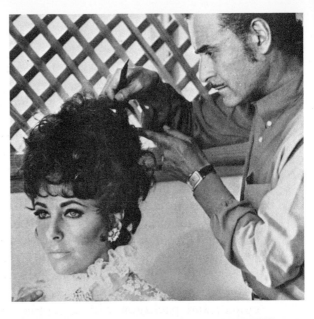

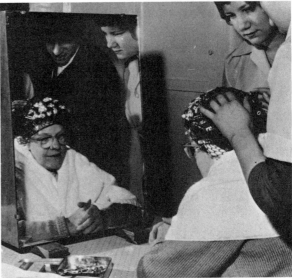

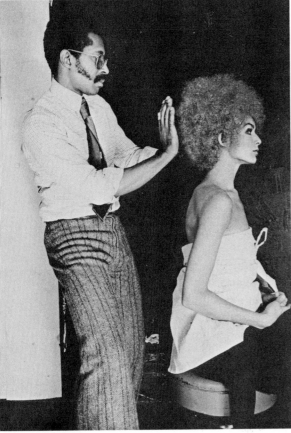

Hairdressing today. Top left, Antoîne, one of the artist-hairdressers who continue the tradition established by Champagne and Léonard, proposes a new style for one of the wealthy clients of his Paris salon. Top right, Alexandre of Paris puts the finishing touches to a new coiffure for movie star Elizabeth Taylor. Left, a black hairdresser creates an Afro-Asian style on a white model. Above, "senior citizens" act as models for apprentice hairdressers at a British training school.

and in England costs £170 (about $400); the regrooming, which takes only one hour, costs £10 ($24) each time. So it is expensive, and it is still experimental. Trichologists are waiting to see if the strain of holding up the new hair accelerates further hair loss.

The designs of the modern wig industry upon men are not limited to head hair. In America in 1968, Lisa Wigs had enormous success when they placed on the market a set consisting of sideburns, a thin moustache, and a small, neat beard, retailed at between 180 and 200 dollars. Men condemned to be conventionally clean-shaven at work could rush home to their instant, swinging sideburns for leisure wear. Other young hopefuls even bought Tarzan chest wigs for that unbuttoned virile look.

A profitable sideline for the wig business has been the manufacture of false eyelashes. Made from natural or synthetic hair and treated in the same way as hair for wigs, they are hand tied to a nylon thread, cut, shaped, curled, and packaged with a supply of glue. They are widely used by young women and by some sophisticated older ones, and there is evidence that American men are now starting to wear them.

In general, recent years have seen a trend toward unisex, and the social implications of this have been discussed in previous chapters. Where hair is concerned it has found expression not merely in similar styles for both sexes and increasing male interest in hair cosmetics, but in unisex hairdressing salons. That old villain, "the demon barber," would no doubt be flattered to find his name commemorated in one of London's first and most famous unisex salons, simply called Sweeney's. There, pop music plays loudly enough to have drowned the cries of the earlier Sweeney's victims, but the current customers, many from the fashion and pop scene (one is singer Mick Jagger), have no complaints. Sweeney's subscribe to the modern cult for hair—long, natural, clean, and well-cut—but they still use Culpepper's herbal shampoo, and a herbal conditioner originally made for Queen Victoria.

So how far has hairdressing really advanced in this scientific age? We have seen how in the Middle Ages the care of the scalp was left in the hands of quacks and charlatans. This situation continued up to the beginning of the present century. During the 18th and 19th centuries, France was the chief center for elixirs: it exported to the USA vast quantities of *Eau de Ninon de L'Enclos* (named after a beautiful courtesan who preserved her hair to the age of 90). But many so-called cures contained dangerous ingredients such as sulfur and mercury, and the great French scientist Lavoisier campaigned unsuccessfully in the 18th century for some control of their contents. One hair tonic, *Eau de Chine,* contained a dangerous solution of silver that drove a woman who used it to the point of madness. In England, Paste of the Sultans, Aurora's Lotion, Spring Dew, were hair lotions with names as unlikely as their contents. In the 19th century, Macassar oil became the rage. Even Byron referred to it, in *Don Juan*:

> In virtues nothing earthy could surpass her
> Save thine "incomparable oil," Macassar!

and chair-backs had to be protected with coverings called antimacassars. The New World became an avid customer for these oils, and it was success in peddling them from door to door that largely laid the foundation of the Rockefeller fortune.

France was renowned for elixirs. Meanwhile, the English experimented with electricity—it could hardly be expected that the invention in the middle of the 18th century of a machine to produce static electricity would be ignored by the hair opportunists. An Englishman, Bartlett, cashed in on it by attaching a glass rod to the generator, and persuading gullible clients

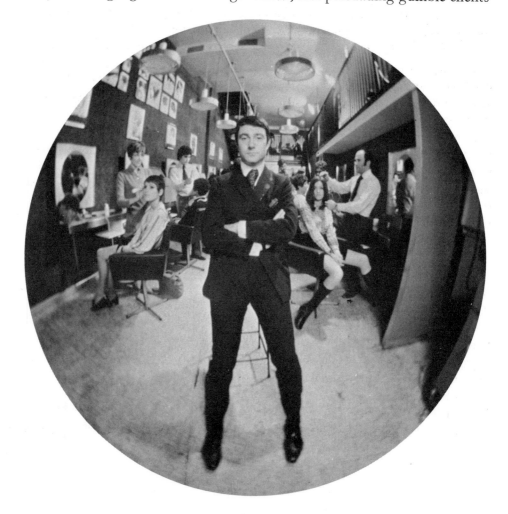

that the resultant prickling sensation in the scalp, and hair standing on end, betokened actual growth. James Graham went even further by opening his so-called Temple of Apollo by the river Thames in London. Here, he claimed to cure every disease by electricity, and several halls were devoted especially to the care of hair. To us now, it may seem absurd, but electricity was the new wonder of the age. One section in the Temple contained an enormous electrified bed, guaranteed to cure frigid women. People credulous enough to believe *that* were not going to query the ability of this new force to preserve hair, although they must have been puzzled when the inventor himself died completely bald at the age of 40, just after publishing his system for preserving hair and living to be 200.

It was only at the end of the last century that serious research into hair health commenced. Undoubtedly the biggest advance has been the modern understanding of scalp hygiene. In the past, hair washing was a rare and erratic business, largely because of the lack of adequate facilities—good soap and hot water. Wigs, powders, and perfumes made a valiant attempt to conceal the dirt and vermin that affected the scalp. But once wigs and powder were abandoned, care of natural hair received a new impetus, and the medical profession at last began to show interest.

The first genuine doctor to get involved with hair since the Middle Ages was an Anglo-Frenchman, Dr. Brown-Séquart, famous for his attempts to rejuvenate patients with juices from the sexual glands of monkeys. At the end of the last century, he devised a special lotion made from female urine, which he claimed would cure baldness. It was hardly a propitious start for medical science in the realm of hair, but it led the way to more serious research. At the St. Louis Hospital in Paris, Sabouraud, a dermatologist, began work that was to establish the principle of disinfection of the scalp, to demonstrate the dangers of harsh soaps, and to lay the foundations for the specialized hair cosmetics industry of today.

Biologists examined hair under the microscope, and learned much about its structure. In 1912, Jackson and McMurtry in the USA published a treatise entitled *Diseases of the Hair,* based on serious medical research. Gradually, a new branch of medical science, called "trichology," has become established, devoted entirely to the study of disorders of the hair and scalp. These disorders, even common dandruff, can now be medically treated. Where these have been contributory factors causing baldness, considerable progress has been made in curing it. But for ordinary male pattern baldness a cure remains elusive.

There is, however, a new move afoot to prevent its onset, arrest its progress, and even produce regrowth. The method is based on the

Vidal Sassoon, who rose from hairdresser's assistant to become one of the wealthiest and most sought-after of international hairdressers, in his New Bond Street, London, salon. Sassoon numbers movie stars, pop idols, and members of the jet set among his clientele and has created hair styles that have been copied by thousands of women.

importance to the scalp of good circulation, and aims at restoring or improving this by ensuring complete scalp hygiene, providing local stimulation to the scalp, and improving general health. Obviously, correct diet and regular shampooing are the first steps. Then, local stimulation is achieved by massage, chemicals, and electrical treatment. But all claims are treated with caution by most trichologists. Their caution seems well justified in view of the number of bald heads in their own profession.

This is the age of the transplant and it seems inevitable that someone had to try transplanting hair. This can be done, but it is expensive, tedious, and moderately painful. A New York dermatologist, Norman Orentreich, has developed a technique of removing "plugs" of live hair from the back of the patient's neck and replanting them on the bald spot from which similar-sized "punches" of skin have been removed in readiness. The process takes four weeks and is costly (around 3000 dollars). Frank Sinatra is numbered among the famous who have undergone this treatment.

Beside these achievements of modern medicine, it seems slightly incongruous to mention the safety razor. And yet this simple gadget has probably contributed more to the sum total of human comfort and convenience than far more intricate inventions. For the very expression "clean-shaven" was for centuries a complete misnomer for a painfully acquired bristly stubble. The cut-throat razor, well-stropped, finally achieved a good shave, but it needed skillful if not professional handling. In 1895, an American, Gillette, invented the safety razor and at last men could shave themselves regularly and easily, leaving the barbers to concentrate for the most part on cutting hair and trimming beards and moustaches. In 1961, the British company Wilkinson Sword produced coated stainless steel blades claimed to give four times more shaves, and in the early 1960s ordinary shaving soaps gave way to aerosol lathers. But meanwhile, electric razors had arrived. In 1969, they were being used by 37 per cent of the male shaving population of the United Kingdom, and by 65 per cent in the United States.

Parallel with the improvements in medical knowledge about hair and technical advances in shaving, came new mechanical techniques for hair styling. The first, in the 1870s, was discovered by a poor, and at the time rather unsuccessful, Parisian hairdresser, Marcel Grateau. He was one day using a curling iron to try to make a lock of his mother's hair, which was hanging straight, match the rest of her naturally wavy hair, when he found that by turning the gently heated iron upside down, he could create the desired effect. To begin with, he had to persuade clients to let him make the new *ondulations,* as they were called, free of charge, but after a move to a new shop near the Théâtre Français, in Paris, and patronage by the famous actress Jane Hading, the new technique caught on, and the demand was so great that clients outbid each other for his services. Marcel was able to retire, wealthy and successful, at the age of 45. He escaped the fate of his predecessors Champagne and Legros and died in his bed at the age of 84.

The Marcel wave, as it was eventually called, went on being popular well into the 1920s, but another breakthrough was just around the corner. It started in 1906 with an announcement in the *Hairdressers' Journal*:

"Mr. C. Nestle, 245 Oxford Street, W.1. begs to invite leading hairdressers to inspect and judge a lady's hair waved permanently by his newly invented and greatly improved process of waving to withstand water, shampoo and all atmospheric influences. Every investigation allowed."

It was the beginning of the permanent wave, a technique that changed the whole concept of hair styling. The inventor, born Karl Ludwig Nessler, was the son of a German shoemaker. He took up hairdressing only because his sight was too poor for him to follow his father's trade. He soon became successful, learning Marcel waving in Paris, but he also experimented with his own ideas. He set up hairdressing salons in London in 1902 (when he changed his name to Charles Nestle) and later in New York.

That first permanent wave was produced by an overhead machine with heavy, heated curlers that dangled like some strange octopus. It was an endurance test for the client, taking up to 10 hours to wave a whole head.

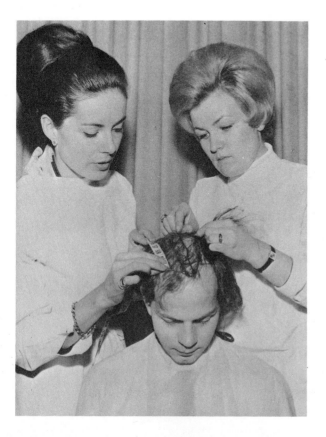

There is still no known cure for ordinary male pattern baldness; the hair loss can be disguised, but not remedied. Hair weaving, which involves threading new, carefully matched hairs onto the remaining natural hair, is one answer. It is the halfway house between wearing a toupee and undergoing a series of hair transplants. Its advantage is that, unlike a wig, it can in all situations be treated exactly like its owner's real hair. Its disadvantage is that it has to be retightened about every two months as the natural hair to which it is attached grows out.

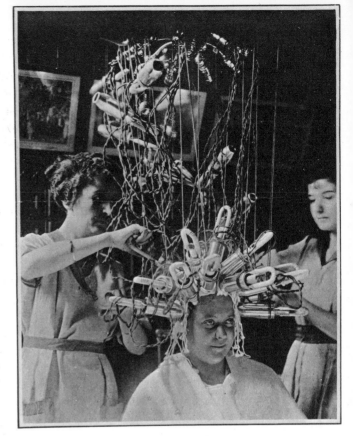

Nestle's first permanent waving machine. Although the original clumsy process was soon superseded, the principle of permanent waving remains unchanged to this day. All permanent waving involves changing the internal structure of the hair, either by heat or by chemical action. The sulfur bonds that hold the hair form are broken. While they are broken the hair is wound around a curler. When the bonds are reconstituted by a "neutralizer," they act to retain the hair in its new shape.

All the same, it produced waves that would last for months and defy wind, weather, and washing. Although the original, clumsy process was soon superseded, the principle has remained the same.

Many variations on the process have since been developed, including do-it-yourself home permanents, and prices have been reduced so much that permanents are available in one form or another to most women in the West. A survey in England in 1969 estimated that 27 per cent of all women had had a professional permanent, 13 per cent a home permanent, and 4 per cent both. Women between the ages of 35 and 64 had more professional permanents than any other age group.

The introduction in the USA in the late 1950s of large wire-mesh rollers for setting the hair could not, at first sight, have appeared very revolutionary—curling hair over heated bits of clay pipe was, after all, an old idea. But these wire rollers demolished the old hairdressing tradition of skill and long training. A rash of new salons sprang up, and partially qualified, or even totally unqualified, hairdressers began back-combing to give the bouffant look that was the order of the day.

The other great recent technical advance has been in hair coloring. Dyes and bleaches, as we have seen, have been used throughout history, but only in this century has the cosmetic chemist devised products that are versatile, controllable, safe, and efficient. Colors can be permanent or temporary, combined with shampoos, or used as rinses. One French firm makes 254 different hair colors. In Great Britain alone, 20 nationally advertised brands shared in 1968 a market with a retail turnover of £9 million ($22 million), and in the same year it was estimated that 6 million women used home bleaches or tints. A feature in the American magazine *Cosmopolitan* in June 1960 marked the passing of the mousy blonde and even the platinum blonde in favor of Just Peachy, Copper Blaze, White-Minx, Chocolate Kiss, Fuchsia, Fury, Frivolous, Fawn, or perhaps Tickled Pink, while noting that "dear old gray-haired granny" had turned Night Silver, True Steel, Silver Blue, Mink, or Smoky Pearl.

Today, bleaches, tints, rinses, shampoos, conditioners, restorers, setting lotions, and hair sprays are marketed in bewildering variety. Many are designed as do-it-yourself products, so safe and simple to use that the last decade has seen a resurgence of home hairdressing, especially among the young. Inexpensive hand hair-driers and even stand driers for use in the home have also played their part, but it is the vogue for simple, natural styles that has most threatened the professional hairdresser.

Fortunately for the industry, only the really young or the really glamorous can get away with long, loose hair, and short natural styles still demand frequent skilled cutting. So although the do-it-yourself trend has undoubtedly worried the professionals, both the increased emphasis on good cutting and the need of the mature woman for more sophisticated styles have ensured that hairdressing is still big business.

But there is still much more to a visit to the hairdresser's than meets the eye. There is the balm of someone caring for you, even if you are paying for it: the luxury of being pampered and maybe even flattered. Most of all, there is the pull of the "confessional," stronger than ever in an age when women are struggling with their new role in an increasingly complex society. The priest is out of fashion, the doctor too busy, but the hairdresser is still there to play the part of confidant. The perfumed intimacy of the salon is exactly right, yet so safely proscribed. The touch is tender, yet the extent of physical contact discreetly limited. The good hairdresser is also a good psychologist, aware that women come not just for a renewal of glamour but for a renewal of spirit and confidence.

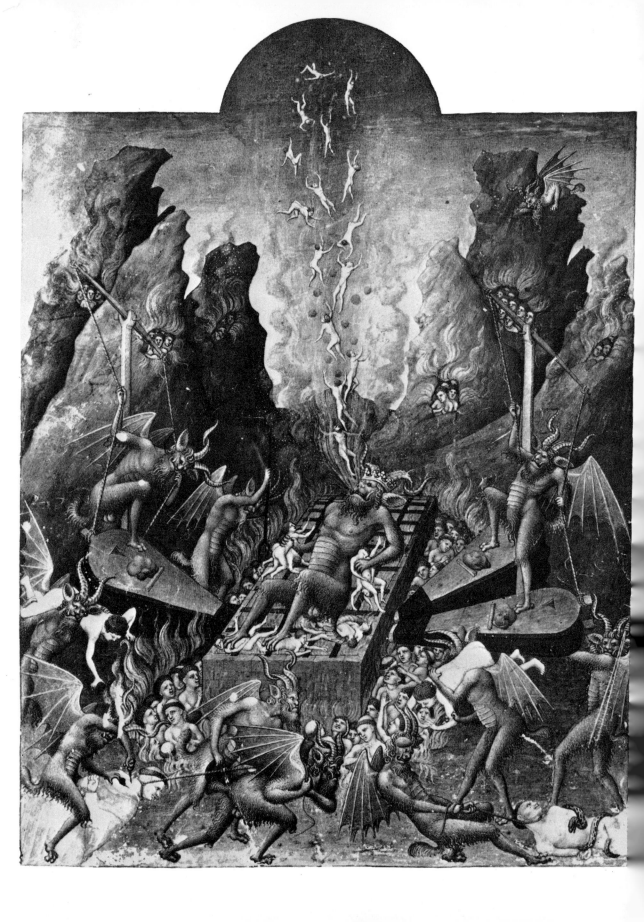

7 Good and Evil

There is no mystery about the age-old link between hair and physical and sexual power. It stems quite naturally, as we have already seen, from the close association of hair with puberty, and from hair's own power of regeneration. But the link between hair and spiritual and magical power is slightly more complex. It involves a two-way shuttle—from man to his gods, and back again to man, drawing in legendary folk heroes on the way. What man most admired in other men, he expected to find in his gods. So he endowed his deities with those human signs of strength and power—flowing locks and beards. And the half-human, half-divine folk heroes who emerged in myth and legend inherited from gods and men hair touched with divinity and possessed of magical power.

The process can be seen perhaps most clearly in relation to one of the first deities of all, the sun. Primitive man's instinctive worship of the sun seems much easier to understand than his devotion to many later and more repulsive gods. These, although they had a few of man's most glorious attributes, had even more of his failings. As a result, they not only complicated their own divine lives with the jealousies and intrigues of celestial power politics, but through their loves, lusts, and cruelties tended to create a hell rather than a heaven upon earth. But the sun was different. To primitive eyes, watching the great golden orb swinging up each day over the rim of the world, it must have seemed the very visitation of a god. And it was a god who brought light to a world of darkness, and warmth to a world of coldness, and who in some strange way nurtured the seeds of life itself. And of course, this god, this sun, had hair. It could be seen. When the glorious face, too bright to gaze upon, was hidden—in the very moment that it slipped behind a cloud, and again just as it emerged—the

Hairy devils and fiends receive sinners consigned to the flames of hell in "The Last Judgement," one of the paintings from the 15th-century illuminated prayer book Les Très Heures du Duc de Berry.

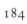

184

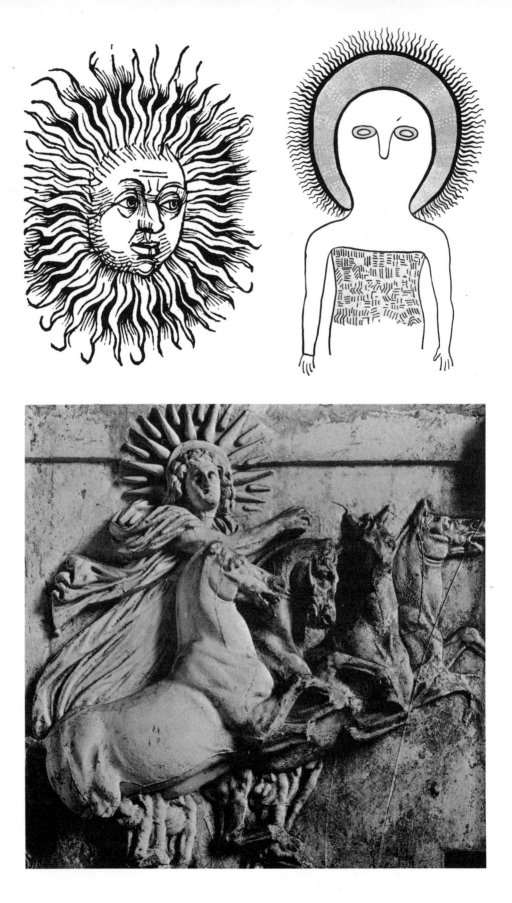

separate rays of shining hair became visible, looking like locks of golden or auburn hair radiating in long dishevelment from a human head.

Small wonder that the early Aryan settlers of India who worshiped the sun addressed their god as "the long-haired," or "the golden-haired," or that ancient hymns of the Hindu sacred book, the *Rig-Veda,* describe the solar god as "the brilliant sun with flaming hair." The same luxuriant locks adorned other sun-gods—the Rhodian Helios, the Greek Apollo, and the Gaulish Cunobelin. Far away across the world, the Mexicans called their sun-god Quetzalcoatl, "bushy-haired," and the Aztecs of Central America styled their god of the declining day Tzontemoc, "of the abundant hair," which describes the long slanting rays of the sun in the evening. The same idea permeated Celtic legend. The 18th-century scholar James Macpherson, in his fraudulent translations of ancient Gaelic epics, made Ossian, the third-century Celtic warrior and bard, lament: "Never more shall I see thy face spreading thy waving golden hair in the East on the face of the clouds." In the Isle of Skye, *grugach,* meaning hairy, is still used today as a name for the sun.

The Romans, too, depicted their sun-god as rich in hair. The poet Claudian, who lived about A.D. 400, invoked him to "scatter daylight abroad with more copious locks," and Roman nurses, according to Tertullian, lulled wakeful children with stories about "the combs of the sun." The ancient Egyptian solar deity, Ra, was adorned "with golden locks." The vital importance of hair in the whole concept is perhaps most clearly shown in an incantation from the *Rig-Veda,* pronounced by the sorcerer-priest when he communed with the fire-god, Agni:

> The hair bears the fire, the hair bears the philtre,
> The hair bears the sky and the earth,
> The hair is the sun which allows us to see the universe.
> All hail to hair!

Solar hair was often depicted as seven distinct locks or rays, a number that probably had planetary significance. Numerous representations of sun-gods from widely different cultures used this idea. Pliny described the colossal figure of the sun made by the first-century Greek artist Zenodorus as having seven such beams, each of them 22½ feet long. A Pompeian wall painting shows Helios with his head encircled by seven well-defined rays, and the Persian sun-god Mithras had, in addition to abundant hair, the same seven beams issuing from his head like spikes. Early Christian art sometimes shows the figure of Christ with seven solar rays around his head. A stylized version of this came to form the halo, and in the temporal sphere was the origin of the crown as a symbol of sovereignty.

Top left, the face of the sun, seen as a human head with hair forming the sun's life-giving rays. Top right, an Australian cave painting probably also represents a sun god. Bottom, a Greek relief of Helios the sun god driving his four-horsed chariot across the skies.

And so hair took on a touch of divinity. From its earthly, human origins, and associations with sexual power, it became a symbol of the magical and spiritual power of the gods. And this power was later reversed from gods back to men as the solar heroes evolved in myth and folklore, and over the centuries became merged and inextricably intermixed with a number of part legendary, part historical figures.

Always, these solar heroes, along with their splendid heads of hair, possessed enormous physical strength, sexual prowess, and magical power—all of which waned if the hair was cut off, like the power of the sun when its rays disappeared over the horizon. Also like the sun, the sun-heroes were solitary figures, walking alone.

The best known of them all is the biblical Samson, whose name may well be derived from the Hebrew word *shemesh*, meaning hair. Samson was a swashbuckling adventurer whose courage and superhuman strength made him the champion of Israel against the Philistines. His downfall came when he became besotted with the faithless Delilah, who was bribed by the Philistine leaders to find out "wherein his great strength lieth, and by

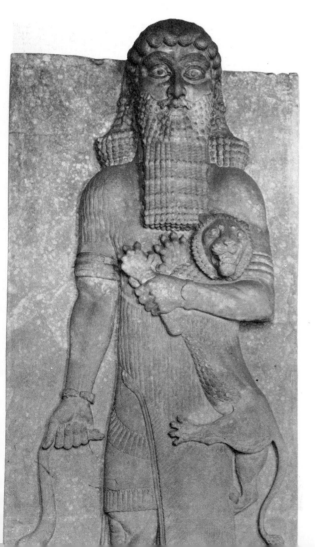

Left, an 8th-century B.C. bas-relief from Khorsabad of the Assyrian sun-hero Gilgamesh. The Gilgamesh legend has many points in common with that of the Greek Hercules, who also slew a lion with his bare hands and was also represented as a muscular, bearded figure.

Right, the beard of Fath Ali, Shah of Persia (1797-1834), was said to be the admiration and delight of his people. It was the beard of kingship in its most luxuriant form, but its glossy blackness conveys menace as well as majesty. In Michelangelo's sculpture (far right) of Moses, in the Church of San Pietro in Vinculi in Rome, completed in 1516, the equally luxuriant beard is of a different kind. It is the beard of wisdom and paternalism, the beard of the prophetic leader.

what means we may prevail against him." After much prevarication Samson was eventually seduced into telling Delilah the truth: "if I be shaven, then my strength will go from me, and I shall become weak, and be like any other man." So Delilah "made him sleep upon her knees; and she called for a man, and she caused him to shave off the seven locks of his head; and she began to afflict him, and his strength went from him." The Philistines were then able to capture Samson easily enough. They put out his eyes and "brought him down to Gaza and bound him with fetters of brass; and he did grind in the prison house." But Samson's shaved hair began to grow again and his strength to return. Soon he was able to tear down the supporting pillars of the house to which his captors had brought him in order to mock and humiliate him. He died with his enemies in the ruins.

But Samson is not the original sun-hero. The true archetype is Gilgamesh of Babylonian legend. Gilgamesh, it is thought, may have been a real historical figure, a conqueror of the Euphrates Valley in the third millennium B.C., who was later given the attributes of a solar deity. His most

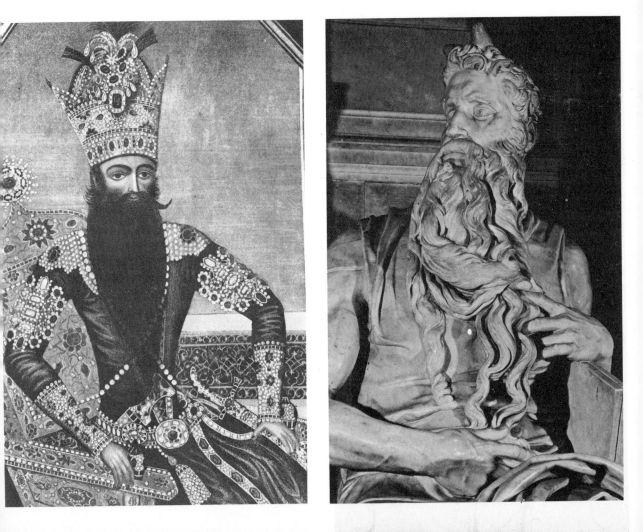

conspicuous features were luxuriant hair down to his shoulders, and a long beard. Sculptures traditionally depict him with long, thick hair clustered into snaky twists. With his mighty sinews, and a half-throttled lion gripped under one arm, he was the prototype both of the Greek Hercules and of the biblical Samson.

The Babylonians believed that, after the seventh month of the year, the sun became enfeebled by a leprous disease that caused its hair to fall out. And so, in the legend, Gilgamesh grows sick at that same time. Like the sun, he is forced to undertake a long journey over dark waters to purify himself so that "the hair of his head is restored," and with it his strength. Like the sun, he returns radiant and refreshed. (The same idea is seen in the saga of the Irish sun-hero, Cuchulainn, who falls ill on the eve of November, at the start of the dark season, and to restore himself sets out for the other world of Labraith's Isle.)

Like Samson, Gilgamesh owed his misfortune to the seductions of a woman, Ishtar, whom he had slighted, and who afflicted him with a loathsome disease that caused his hair to fall out. There are obvious implications of venereal disease in these old legends. It must be more than coincidence that the Aztec word *nanahuatl,* meaning "afflicted with venereal disease," is also a name given to their sun-god. Certainly the sun-heroes, such as Hercules and Samson, were sexual adventurers, and the ancient link between hair and virility echoes in their exploits. In the *Rig-Veda* the sun itself is described as "the suitor of maidens, the husband of wives," and a Hebrew psalm describes the rising sun "as a bridegroom coming out of his chamber."

Not only the sun-gods, but many others, were distinguished by long hair and a beard, which symbolized their strength and power. Zeus and Poseidon in Greek Mythology, Jupiter and Neptune in Roman, and Thor and Odin in Norse—these and a hundred more were hairy, or bearded, or both. Even Jehovah was traditionally represented with a beard.

Thor, the powerful Norse god of thunder, was usually depicted not merely bearded but red-bearded, which represented the fiery appearance of the lightning he could hurl. Here was a god who certainly made full use of his beard, shaking it when roused, and speaking into it to make everyone quail. His anger was described in his bristling hair and tossing beard, and a rather nasty habit of letting his brows sink down over his eyes. When Thor met King Olaf of Norway in the 10th century, at a time when Christianity was encroaching on his cult, he "blew hard into his beard, and raised his beard's voice," which clearly did not stop Christianity but did produce a very unpleasant storm.

Opposite, the prophet Abraham, from the fresco by Filippino Lippi (c. 1457-1504) in the Church of S. Maria Novella in Rome. Although artists tended to portray biblical characters in the fashions of their own times, certain traditions became fixed. A clean-shaven Hebrew prophet is almost unthinkable. Overleaf, in Agostino di Duccio's 15th-century bas-relief of cherubim in water, hair and water mingle their textures so that the fine hair of purity echoes the waves of the cleansing waters. On p. 191: in the painting Dead Poet *carried by a* Centaur *by Gustave Moreau (1826-98), the hairy animal body of the centaur symbolizes the bestial side of man's nature and contrasts with the smooth skin of the poet, who represents the idealistic, imaginative side.*

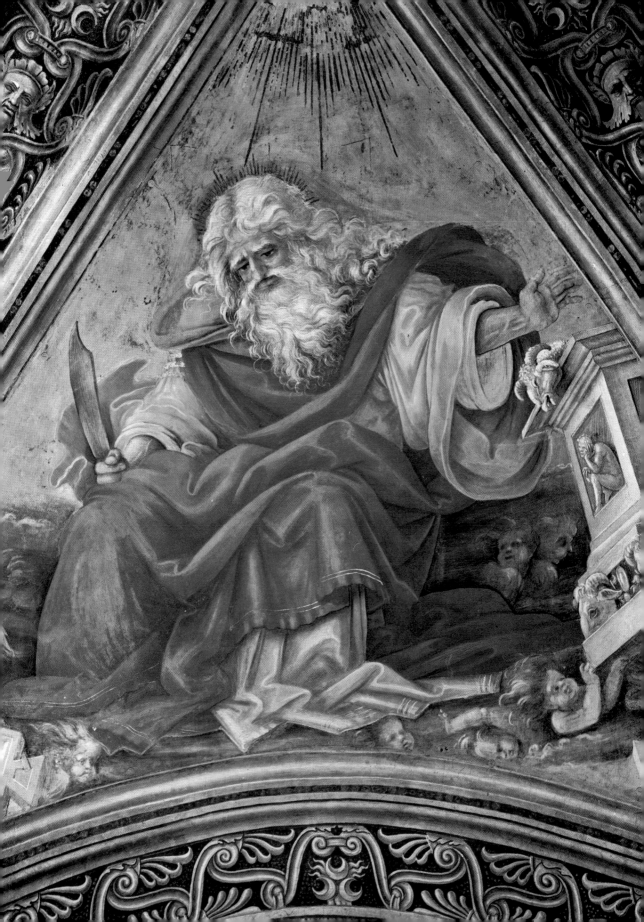

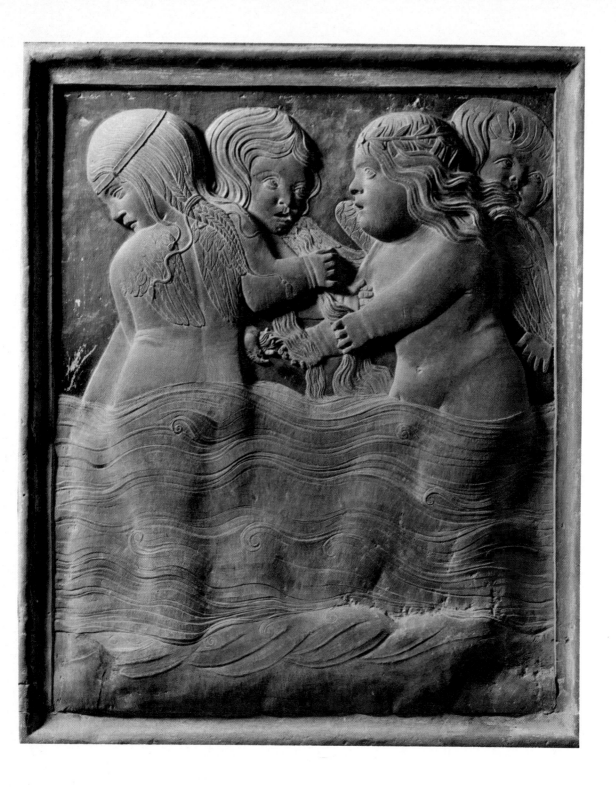

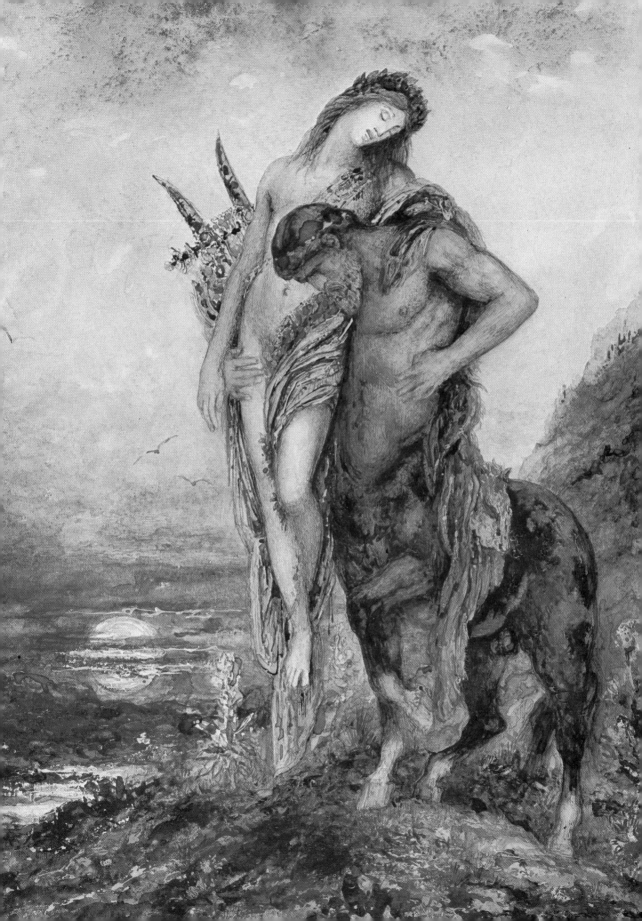

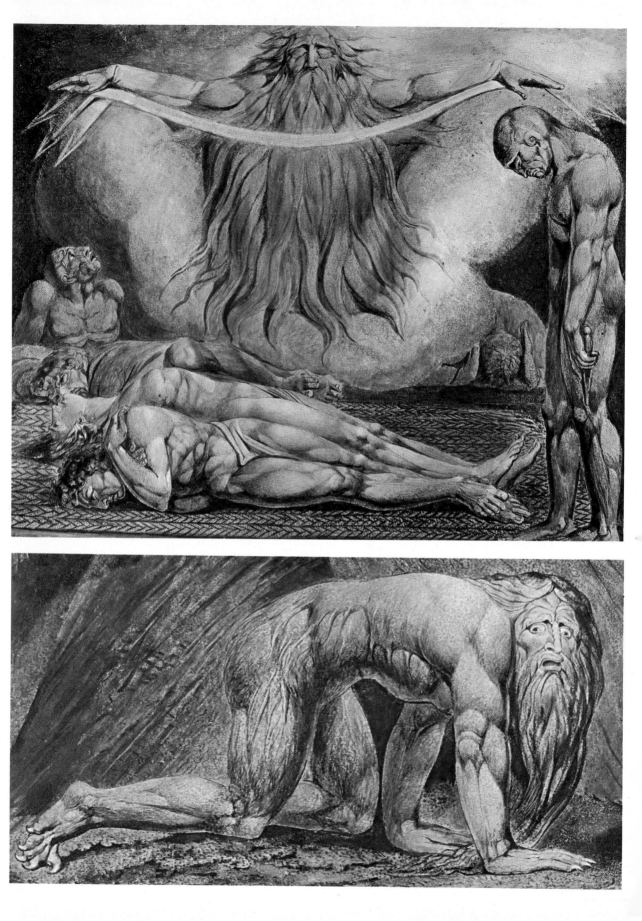

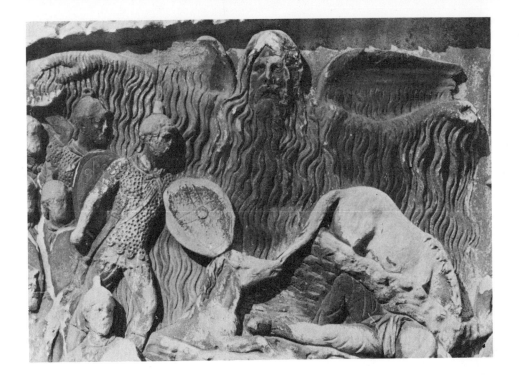

To many people the beard has been considered sacred. Mohammed kept his unshorn and his followers had to do the same. To swear by the beard of the prophet was, and still is among orthodox Moslems, the greatest oath of all. Even the traditional nursery tales of children hint at the ancient idea of the oath upon the beard:

Little pig, little pig, let me come in!

No, no, by the hair of my chinny, chin, chin!

Like the beards of gods and prophets, the beards of kings have been reckoned particularly sacred and important to the realm. At one time it was believed that three hairs from a French king's beard, secured under the wax seal on a document, assured the fulfillment of the promises made therein. The ancient kings of Persia, Nineveh, Assyria, and Babylon were all traditionally depicted with beards, and for state occasions the normally smooth-chinned Egyptian kings (not to mention some Egyptian queens) assumed the royal dignity of false beards.

Because of the beard's dignity and sacred nature, it has at certain periods of history been a gross insult to tamper with it—to cut it, to pull it, or even, in some countries, to touch it. The Bible tells of the bloody vengeance David wreaked upon the Ammonites for the supreme indignity they had inflicted on his servants by cutting off one half of each man's beard. The strictly Orthodox Jew preserves his beard intact to this day, although

Above, a detail from the Column of Marcus Aurelius depicts the rain god Jupiter Pluvius shedding beneficent rain upon the Romans and sweeping their enemies away in a whirling torrent. Left: two paintings by William Blake (1757-1827). In The House of Death *(top) the bearded figure of Adam extends protecting arms over the sick in a leper house. Bottom,* Nebuchadnezzar, *who "did eat grass like oxen" and whose "hairs were grown like eagles' feathers."*

surprisingly the *Jewish Encyclopedia* now insists that the reason is "that God gave man a beard to distinguish him from woman and that it is therefore wrong to antagonize nature." This seems an odd rationalization of ancient beliefs concerning the sanctity of hair.

Earlier ages had not yet come to doubt their superstitions about hair. They had a legacy of so many stories that seemed to confirm its magical power. In Greek myth, there is the story of Nisus, the king who possessed among his gray hairs one glittering purple lock, which was a talisman that kept safe his city of Megara. But when Megara was besieged by Minos, king of Crete, Scylla, the daughter of Nisus, fell in love with her father's enemy and at the dead of night stole to her sleeping father's couch and cut off the magic purple lock. Slipping out through the gates of the city to the enemy camp, she presented it to Minos, and so betrayed her father.

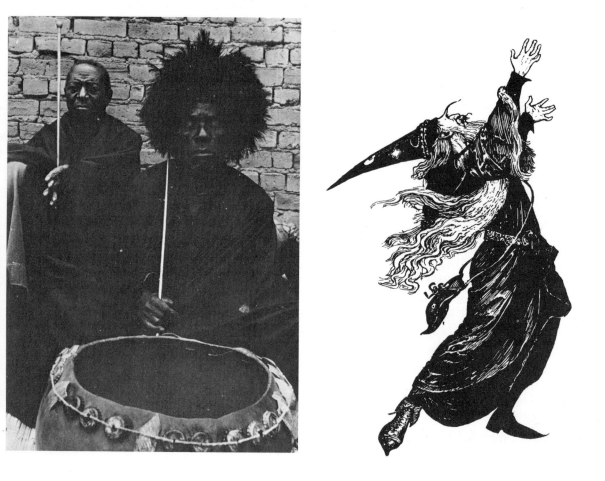

Left the witchdoctor Wafanaka, "voice of the Black God of Rhodesia," used his unkempt, disheveled hair to give him an awe-inspiring appearance and to demonstrate his holiness and his aloofness from everyday worldly trivialities. Right, a traditional white-bearded fairy-tale wizard.

Then there is the story, told by the natives of the island of Nias off the west coast of Sumatra, of a young king, Laubo Maros, whose strength lay in one special hair that grew hard as copper wire. Laubo Maros seduced his uncle's wife, and the injured husband sought the help of the Sultan of Johore. Laubo Maros was captured and successively thrown into the sea, burned on a blazing pyre, and hacked at with swords, but nothing could kill him. In the end he, like Samson, was betrayed by a woman—his wife revealed the fatal secret of the magic hair. When it was plucked out, his strength left him and he was killed.

From this kind of legend, and the fears they both revealed and transmitted, flourished a great crop of superstitions and myths about hair. They found expression not only in relatively harmless ways, such as the Frankish kings being forbidden to cut their hair from childhood, but also in darker deeds. Even the Frankish taboo had its dark side, for in the sixth century, when the wicked brothers Clotaire and Childebert coveted the kingdom of their dead brother Clodomir, they inveigled into their power the two little sons of the dead king. Then they sent a messenger bearing scissors and a naked sword to the children's grandmother, Queen Clotilde, in Paris. The envoy showed her the scissors and the sword, and asked her to choose whether the children should be shorn and live, or remain unshorn and die. To cut their hair would disinherit them from the throne, and the proud queen preferred to see them die. And so they did, murdered by the hand of their ruthless uncle, Clotaire.

Not only kings, but priests, medicine men, sorcerers, and even ordinary people made a point of retaining their hair to preserve to the full the magical strength and power they believed it gave them. According to Frazer, in *The Golden Bough*, Aztec priests were forbidden to cut their hair, at least until they were relieved of their duties in old age. Often it grew so long that its weight became a great burden. Medicine men among the Haida Indians of Queen Charlotte Islands, off British Columbia, might neither cut nor comb their hair, so that it was not only long but also tangled. Priests of the Hos, a negro tribe of Togo in West Africa, were forbidden to use a razor and, before trimming their hair, had to seek permission from their god, whose seat the hair was supposed to be. Sorcerers of the Masai clan of the El Kiboron in East Africa, who believed they possessed the art of rain-making, would not pluck a single hair from their beards for fear of losing their magic power.

Men of the Tsetsaut tribe of British Columbia thought that if they cut their hair, they would grow old quickly. In the island of Ceram, in the East Indies, men believed that to be shorn would make them so weak and enervated that they would lose their wives. The same idea persisted in the Timorlaut Islands of Indonesia, where only widowers and men on a journey were allowed to cut their hair, if they offered a fowl or pig in sacrifice first. Male Malays were forbidden to cut their hair during their wife's pregnancy and for 40 days after the child was born. Among the Alfoors of Celebes, an island in the Malay archipelago, the priest who looked after the ricefields might not cut his hair during the period beginning a month before the rice was sown and ending after it had been harvested.

Hair has often been left uncut until some vow has been fulfilled, in order to confer extra strength for the task. Frazer quotes the example of 6000 Saxons who "once swore they would not poll their hair nor shave their beards until they had taken vengeance on their foes." In ancient Egypt, where the whole head was normally shaved, it was the custom for those undertaking a journey to allow the hair to grow and remain uncut until they turned homeward. The same idea is found in widely separated parts of the world, embracing both peaceful and warlike expeditions.

Right across the world, from east to west, belief in a connection between the hair and the soul has left its mark on many different cultures. North American Indians thought that the hair imprisoned the soul, and that by scalping an enemy they captured the soul and prevented it from escaping and returning to seek its revenge. Possession of the scalp also, of course,

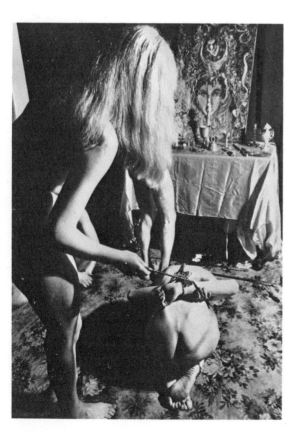

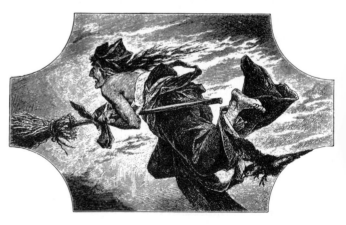

Above, the common conception of a witch—an ugly, hairy, skinny old hag on a broomstick. Her hairiness was the hairiness of evil, derived from her association with the hairy devil, and much of her power was believed to reside in her hair. So captured witches were often shaved partly or completely to destroy their supernatural power. Present-day witches use their powers only for good—they are "white" or benevolent witches—and their appearance has changed with their purpose. They look no different from ordinary mortals (left) and straggling hair plays no part in their new image.

added to their own stock of magical power. The same basic idea lay behind the ancient Greek belief that until a lock of hair had been given to Proserpina, the goddess of death, she would refuse to release the soul from the dying body. When Dido, the legendary Queen of Carthage, stabbed herself in order to avoid being forced to remarry, she lingered in agony until Juno, the goddess protector of women, sent the messenger Iris to cut off a lock of her hair.

Such widespread faith in the power of hair was bound to find a place in European witchcraft. So potent was hair conceived to be that in Scotland it was ominous even to meet a woman with her head uncovered. If a woman shook her hair at you, anything might happen. One Bessie Skebister was accused and convicted in 1633 of causing a disease in another woman, Margaret Mudie, whose cow had trespassed among her corn, by the simple but deadly expedient of "shaking of her hair." Not surprisingly, when a climax of superstitious fear drove society to the cruelties and excesses of a witch hunt, it was common practice in Europe to shave the wretched suspects before handing them over to the torturers. According to Frazer, in his *Folk-lore in the Old Testament* (1918), it was customary in France to shave the witch's whole body, partly to search for hidden marks of Satanic allegiance, and partly to deprive her of the strength and protection she derived from her hair. Sometimes, so susceptible to suggestion is the human mind, it even seemed to work. Joannes Millaeus, in his *Praxis Criminis*, published in 1541, describes a witch trial in Toulouse at which the accused confessed only after they had been stripped and completely shaved. One woman, who had endured the worst her torturers could devise, confessed at once when her body was shaved. The 15th-century German inquisitor Jacob Sprenger contented himself with shaving only the heads of suspected witches; but his more thorough colleague Cumanus shaved the whole bodies of 41 women before committing them all to the flames.

This practice of shaving witches was not confined to Europe. A British writer, W. Crooke, in his book on *The Folklore of Northern India*, published in 1896, mentions that in the province of Bastar, "if a man is adjudged guilty of witchcraft, he is beaten by the crowd, his hair is shaved, the hair being supposed to constitute his power of mischief.... Women suspected of sorcery have to undergo the same ordeal; if found guilty, the same punishment is awarded, and after being shaved, their hair is attached to a tree in some public place." He also records that among the Bhils of central India, when a woman was convicted of witchcraft, a lock of hair was cut from her head and buried in the ground "that the last link between her and her former powers of mischief might be broken." Among the Aztecs a similar practice was found: the head of a witch was cropped before death to remove all her power of sorcery and enchantment.

The human mind has always conceived of supernatural forces as working for either good or evil. And so hair magic, although strongly associated with divinity and benign power, also has—as we have seen in relation to witchcraft—dark links with malignant forces. Gods and prophets are traditionally bearded, but so are devils, demons, wizards, and even witches. Here, hairiness seems not only to symbolize the maleficent powers these creatures are able to wield, but also to emphasize their bestiality. Whereas man has constantly depicted his gods and heroes as possessing the best features of humanity, he has frequently clothed his evil spirits in the garb of animals.

As the counterpart to the monarch of heaven, the monarch of hell has often been represented with a long beard, although, like Judas's, it is traditionally red to symbolize his evil nature. Pluto, the Greek lord of the underworld, was described by the Italian poet Tasso in the 16th century as having a long beard descending over his chest. The devil's body is frequently hairy—probably an inheritance together with horns and hooves, from the goat-like god Pan and the satyrs of Greek mythology. The demon denizens of the underworld are often depicted covered with hair, as are those worshipers of the devil, the witches. Shakespeare gives beards to the three weird sisters in *Macbeth*:

> . . . you should be women,
> And yet your beards forbid me to interpret
> That you are so.

The association of evil spirits with beast-like qualities is embedded deep in the human psyche, and this association holds true for human beings who by their evil activities have placed themselves outside the pale of human society. Traditionally, werewolves, vampires, and other demon animals have been regarded as human beings in league with the devil, who, in their changed form, prey upon human flesh and blood. The wolf-man seems to be among the very oldest of the dark dreads of mankind. Many different elements have fused together in the course of time to make the werewolf myth so strong that it lingers to this day in some religious rites, and so widespread that it can be found in almost every culture.

One practice that no doubt helped to originate the idea was the use of wolf totems in the worship of dead ancestors, leading to a concept of the dead transformed into a divine sort of superwolf. The notion was confirmed by primitive interpretations of the storm-wind as the rush of dead men's

In most cultures the devil is depicted as hairy. The otherwise rather benign-looking devil on a horse (top left) has a mane of hair to go with his clawed feet; the horned, winged devil (top right) has a hairy tail; the seated devil (bottom left) has no less than three beards. The Romanesque relief (bottom right) shows a woman destroying a devil's power by plucking his head.

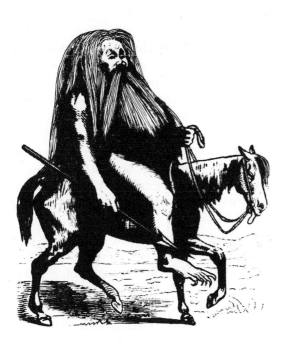

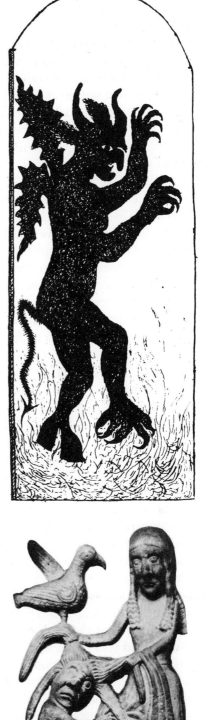

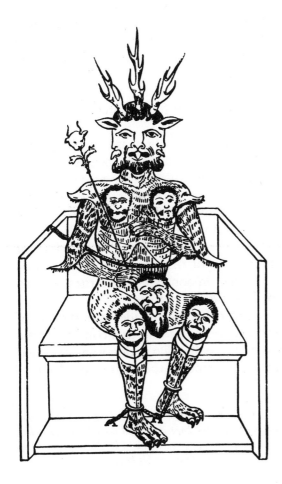

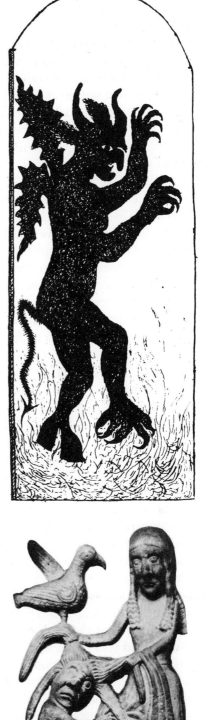

souls, or the howling of wolf-like monsters. Another factor, even further back in the reaches of atavistic memories and fears, may have been the trauma of man's enforced descent from the trees at the time when shrinking forests turned him from a peaceful fruit-picking vegetarian into a carnivorous hunter on the plains. The real experience of primitive man may well have paralleled the allegorical expulsion from Eden, as he learned to hunt in packs and to tear at living flesh, substituting new cunning for old innocence in his effort to survive.

It is possible that this remorseless transition, which made man a killer, lingered on in ancestral memory and later re-emerged in the werewolf myth and in lycanthropy, a form of madness in which the raving patient, believing himself a wolf with lupine teeth, refuses to eat anything but raw and bloody meat. This hysteria can also involve unrestrained sexual attacks, and modern psychiatrists have interpreted it as a throwback to atavistic behavior patterns. Closely linked to the werewolf legend were the wild, war-mad berserkers, northern warriors who dressed in wolves' skins and were said to howl in a wolf-like fashion and to ravage their victims like animals.

The Roman werewolf was commonly called a "skin-changer" or "turn-coat." Medieval legend followed up this idea, believing that while the werewolf kept his human form, his hair grew inward: when he wished to become a wolf, he simple turned himself inside out. In many trials prisoners were closely interrogated about this strange inversion, and some poor creatures were cut up and flayed in an attempt to detect ingrowing hair. Other theories harked back to the berserkers and argued that the possessed person had only to put on a wolf's skin to assume instant lupine form and character.

Indian mythology has its equivalent of the werewolf in the rakshasas, mis-shapen giants with red hair and beards and protruding teeth, who devour human flesh. Their bodies are covered with coarse, bristling hair and their huge mouths hang open as they howl through the woods, lusting after the flesh and blood of men. And so an ancient Hindu myth and the 17th-century European nursery story of Red Riding Hood both carry echoes of the same ancestral fears.

The Chinese—and since, the 11th century, the Japanese—had their equivalent in werefoxes, and in Europe there was a great crop of wolfish gods. The Germanic god Woden chased through stormy nights at the head of his wild pack of wolves, as did the Thracian god Zagreus with his maenads (raving women) clad in fox pelts. From the same bubbling cauldron of legends come the many stories of Bluebeard, briefly meeting

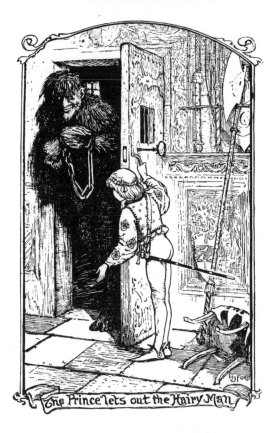

The Prince lets out the Hairy Man

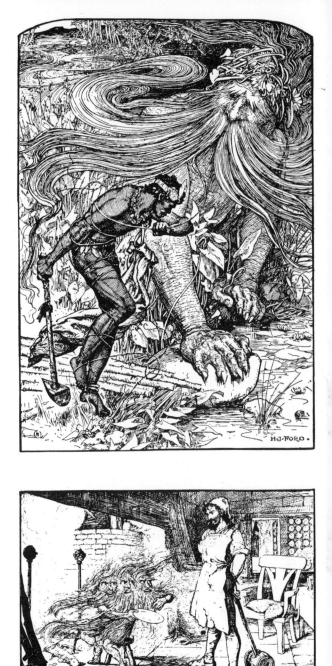

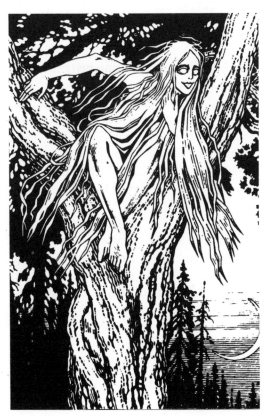

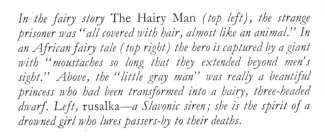

In the fairy story The Hairy Man (top left), the strange prisoner was "all covered with hair, almost like an animal." In an African fairy tale (top right) the hero is captured by a giant with "moustaches so long that they extended beyond men's sight." Above, the "little gray man" was really a beautiful princess who had been transformed into a hairy, three-headed dwarf. Left, rusalka—a Slavonic siren; she is the spirit of a drowned girl who lures passers-by to their deaths.

with reality in the 15th century in the grim form of Gilles de Rais, the French Bluebeard, convicted of torturing, decapitating, or beating to death (to the accompaniment of incredible sexual perversions) no less than 150 children, in homage to Satan.

The fear and fascination of the werewolf dies hard. Localized outbreaks of lycanthropy have occurred in history, notably in France at the end of the 16th and beginning of the 17th century, with gangs of rural poachers terrifying the countryside behind werewolf masks. The very name was nationally resurrected in Germany after World War I in the paramilitary *Organization Werewolf,* and again in Himmler's call in 1945 to harass "like werewolves" the Allied lines of communication in occupied Germany. In Africa, terrorists in the Congo operated in the 1960's as "leopard-men," wearing leopard skins and using iron claws to lacerate their victims. In the religious rites of the Moroccan brotherhood of the "Isawiyya," men still dress up as cats, lions, hyenas, and wolves, and work themselves into a

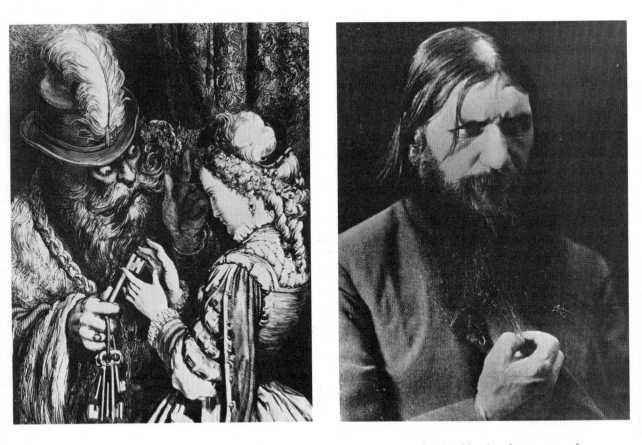

The story of Bluebeard (left), who murdered his wives, makes his blue beard a synonym for corruption and lust. Bluebeard has often been associated—unjustly—with Gilles de Rais, who confessed to monstrous crimes in 15th-century France. Right, Rasputin, another hairy lover accused of nameless crimes.

frenzy by ritual dancing, after which they tear living kids and lambs to pieces with their bare hands.

By contrast the magic and influence of women's hair is traditionally more soft and subtle, but often no less fatal. Just as the sun-gods and heroes underlie myths and superstitions about hair, so do legendary female figures such as Lilith and Medusa.

Lilith was gifted with a marvelous and fatal beauty, and her most compelling feature was her hair. The 19th-century English poet Dante Gabriel Rossetti describes how she brings soft kisses and soft sleep to a young man, but adds the sinister lines:

> Lo! as that youth's eyes burned at thine, so went
> Thy spell through him, and left his straight neck bent,
> And round his heart one strangling golden hair.

Talmudic tradition confused the name Lilith with the word for night, *layah,* and so Lilith became a night demon, who lay with sleeping men, and

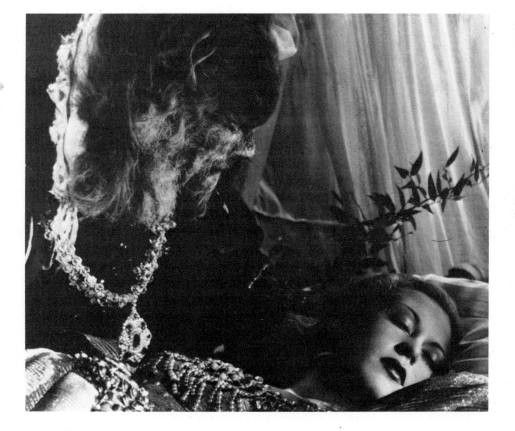

A scene from the Jean Cocteau film Beauty and the Beast *is full of hair symbolism. The "beast" is hairy like an animal—once again to represent man's bestial side, and because hairiness is the sign of the savage and the potential rapist. The "beauty," by contrast, is smooth-skinned, defenselessly feminine, and her hair is the fine, fair hair of purity and innocence.*

204

Just look at him! There he stands,
With his nasty hair and hands.
See! his nails are never cut;
They are grim'd as black as soot;
And the sloven, I declare,
Never once has comb'd his hair;
Any thing to me is sweeter
Than to see Shock-headed Peter.

whose offspring were demons. In this way, medieval Jewry explained wet dreams and nocturnal emissions.

As with the werewolf legend, many different elements have gone to build up myths about the fatal charm of siren tresses. Lilith's own use of potent hair may simply have had its origin in the hairy nature ascribed to all demons. The Medusa legend may have derived in part from this kind of background, and in part also from the general Greek belief in the power of hair. Once beautiful, with many suitors, Medusa was unlucky enough to attract the god Neptune himself, and to yield to his ardors in the very temple of Minerva. That goddess took her vengeance not on Neptune, who was her equal, but on the wretched Medusa, whose glorious hair she turned to scaly serpents, so that its beauty might never tempt god or man again. To make doubly sure, she decreed that anyone who looked upon Medusa's head would be turned to stone. According to Ovid:

> The hissing snakes her foes more sure ensnare,
> Than did they lovers once when shining hair.

Looking at old legends, it seems as if humanity had some inner need to frighten itself. The Greek hero Perseus, protected by the helmet of Pluto (which made him invisible) and armed by the gods, flew on wings borrowed from Mercury to cut off Medusa's head. This may have been the end of Medusa, but it was not the end of the legend. It lived on in the sirens, the Lorelei, the vily, and all the mermaid folktales of different lands.

The vily of Slav legend are beautiful women who have eternal youth so long as they preserve their long fair hair. It they lose a single hair, they die. Any man who sets eyes on one yearns for her from the depths of his soul, so deeply that his longing will eventually kill him. The Lorelei was equally fatal to boatmen on the Rhine who chanced to see her combing her golden hair. Even the cold waters of Lapland were haunted by Akkruva, a water spirit whose head was covered with long hair although the lower part of her body was that of a fish; she, too, sat on rocks, rinsing and combing her hair. The mermaid in British folklore is also a dangerous siren against whose wiles no ship or sailor is safe; her aim is to lure a human being into marriage with her so that she may acquire a soul. And so the ancient tale of Lilith finds its echo in legends that are still half-believed in the remoter parts of Scotland and the Hebrides.

Close relatives of the mermaids and water nymphs, but with feathers instead of hair, are the swan-maidens of Germany. Although they are closely linked with the Teutonic races, they appear also in folklore as far away as Arabia, Japan, East Africa, Polynesia, and South America. In one story of *The Arabian Nights,* a young goldsmith called Hasan discovers

One of the cautionary tales from the German children's book Struwwelpeter *by Dr. Heinrich Hoffmann, first privately published in 1845, illustrates the consequences of neglecting attention to cleanliness and tidiness.*

ten swans in a garden whose door he has been forbidden to unlock. He sees the swans discard their feathers to reveal themselves as beautiful maidens, who plunge into a pool. Enraptured by the perfection of their bodies, he falls instantly in love with one of them, and pines after her until he is told that if he steals her feathers while she is bathing, she will be forced to follow him until she regains them. This plot succeeds and Hasan makes her his wife. Eventually, the maiden discovers the hiding place of her feathers, and flies away to the coast of Borneo. After many adventures, Hasan rediscovers his wife, who in the meanwhile has come to realize how much she loves him, and they live happily ever after. This happy ending is unusual; normally the man smitten with love for a swan-maiden is left to pine to his death.

With such a background in religion, myth, and legend, hair has inevitably become involved in a mass of folk superstition. Perhaps because of the association of red hair with the devil, and with Judas Iscariot who betrayed Jesus, redheads have for centuries had the reputation of being deceitful—and sometimes of being hot-tempered as well. In English folklore, if a woman's hair grows to a point low on the brow, it is said to indicate that she will live to be a widow, and so it is often called a "widow's peak." Similarly if a married woman whose hair is normally straight suddenly develops two curls on her temples, one on each side, it is a sign that her husband has not long to live.

There have been a mass of taboos relating to the washing and cutting of hair, mostly originating in the ancient belief that the soul or spirit dwelt in the head. Obviously, it was important not to disturb it more than necessary. In some cultures—the Burmese, for example—the whole business was undertaken with great solemnity. Fortunately, few people have taken such extreme precautions as the chief of the Namosi of Fiji, who always insisted on eating a man before having his hair cut.

Because a king's hair was considered particularly sacred, it followed that cutting it was particularly hazardous. It was made an affair of state when the king of Cambodia's hair was cropped. Priests placed on the barber's fingers rings set with large stones that were supposed to contain spirits favorable to the king. During the operation the Brahmans struck up with noisy music to drive away the evil spirits. The hair and nails of the mikado, the emperor of Japan, might be cut only while he was asleep, probably because his soul was believed to be absent then from his body, and so could not be hurt by the scissors.

The Maoris believed that cutting the hair could produce thunder and lightning. The same fear may lie behind the traditional belief of sailors that, at sea, hair or nails must be cut only during a storm, when presumably the worst was already happening. Another reason may have been that in desperate situations sailors cut their hair as offerings to the sea-god, and premature cutting might be an ill omen.

The cutting of hair has often been associated with the passing from a taboo state to a normal state. A convert to Islam from an unsanctioned religion was required not only to be washed or anointed with water, but to have his hair cut off. The Bible decreed that the leper, when purified

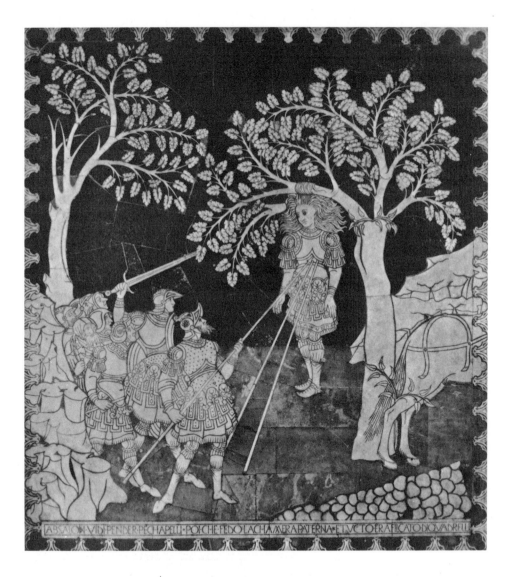

Absalom, son of David, revolted against his father and was killed when he hung helplessly caught by the head in a tree. It is usually assumed that his hair became entangled in a branch, although there is no biblical authority for this. We are told, though, that he had a fine head of hair—"he weighed the hair of his head at two hundred shekels."

of his uncleanness, must shave off his locks, eyebrows, and all the hair of his body. It was a general principle in Rabbinic Judaism that anyone who had become ritually unclean was obliged to cut off his hair. The second-century Greek author Lucian describes how if one of the Galli, the male devotees of the goddess Cybele at her shrine in Hierapolis, saw the corpse of a relative, he became unclean for 30 days, and could not enter the sanctuary. At the end of this period he had to shave his head, after which he was granted access again. In ancient Israel, hair was deliberately allowed to grow during the entire period of festivals and celebrations, and deliberately cut at their conclusion. This cutting of hair symbolized people's return to a state of normality.

The ban on cutting hair during religious festivals led to the association of hair-cutting with the defilement of religious occasions. One old English saying goes:

It was better you were never born
Than on the Sabbath pare hair or horn.

And Friday as well as Sunday came to be commonly considered unlucky for cutting hair and nails, though with local variations. In the county of Northumberland, Friday was unlucky for hair but permissible for nails, and the reverse was true on Sundays. Attempts were made in England to extend superstitious and religious sanction to legal sanction. In 1592 a law was passed fining any barber 10 shillings, which was a large sum in those days, if he profaned the Lord's Day by shaving a single customer, except on the two Sundays preceding or following assize weeks.

Barbers were victims of the law, but others were harassed by fanatical Sabbatarians. There is an anecdote about the Reverend Patrick Brontë, father of the famous novelists, who was reported as having been seen shaving himself on a Sunday morning. The poor man not only denied it, but confessed: "I never shaved myself in all my life, or was ever shaved by anyone else. I have so little beard that a little clipping every three months is all that is necessary." He was obviously embarrassed by such an admission and hoped it would go no further, for he added: "I should like you to keep what I say in your family." So much for pious hopes. Human nature being what it is, the story not only got repeated, but written down to survive to this day.

One of the most powerful reasons for caution on the part of primitive peoples when it came to cutting their hair, was their widely held belief in homeopathic and sympathetic magic. Homeopathic magic involved the production of an effect simply by imitating it, so that in Laos, when an elephant hunter started out, his wife was forbidden to cut her hair, because

Opposite, a 14th-century primitive Italian painting of Saint Mary Magdalen clothes her entirely in her long hair—the hair with which she washed the feet of Jesus Christ. Overleaf: The Gorgon and the Heroes, by Giulio Sartorio (1860–1932). On p. 211; the severed head of Medusa, the most terrible of the three gorgons, painted by Caravaggio (1573–1610).

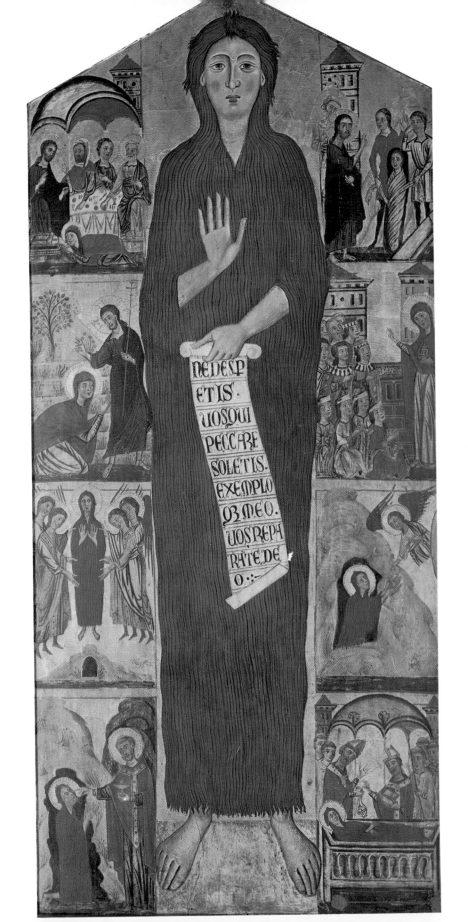

NEDESP
ETIS·
UOSQUI
PECCARE
SOLETIS·
EXEMPLO
OR MEO·
UOSREPA
RÁTE·DE
O ∴•

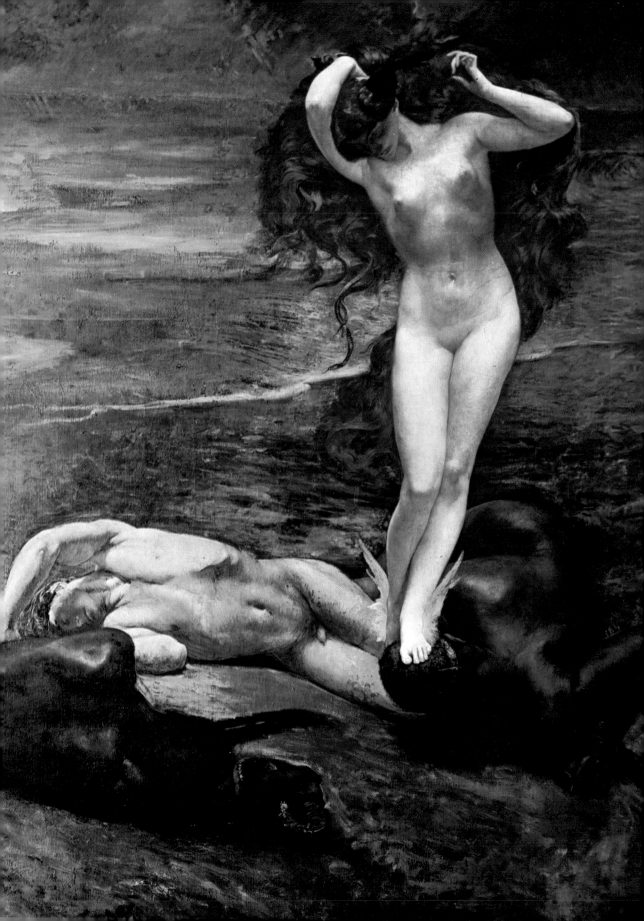

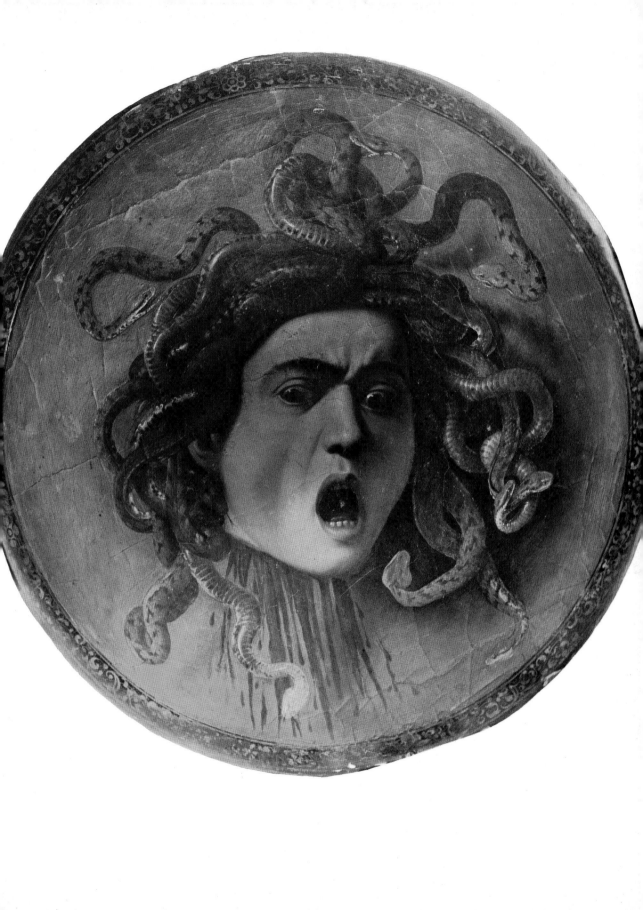

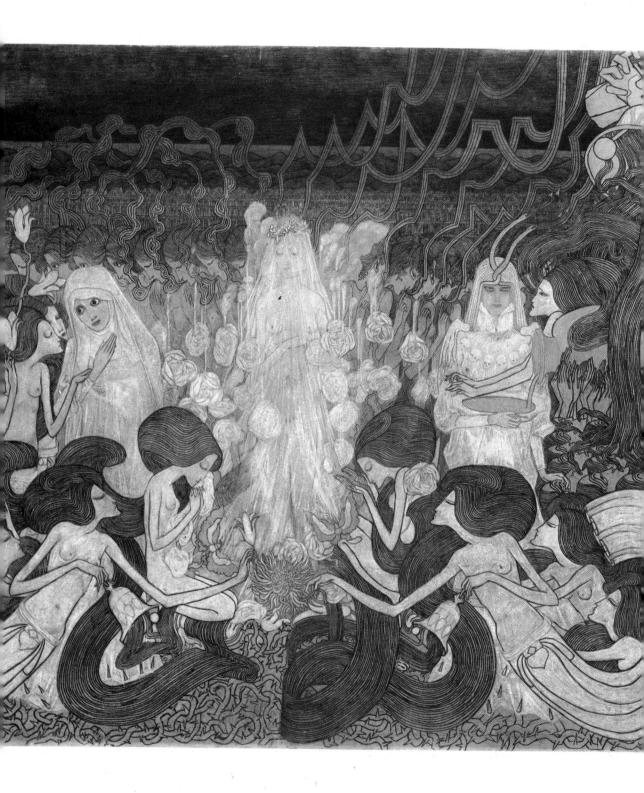

this would enable the elephant to sever any ropes that were used to restrain him. Similarly among the Sea Dyaks of Banting in Sarawak, when a husband was away fighting, a wife could not oil her hair, or her husband would be prone to slip. Among some Singhalese, the hair of a woman in labor, and that of her husband, was left unbound to ensure an unobstructed birth. The same idea was used in some fertility rites; in Mexico during the ancient festival in honor of the goddess of maize, known as "the long-haired mother," the women had to wear their hair unbound, and shake and toss it as they danced, so that the tassels of maize would grow in profusion.

Sympathetic magic involved the belief that any part of the body, when severed, retained some sort of connection with its owner. If a magician or sorcerer should manage to gain possession of the severed portions—be they hair or nail clippings, or even items of clothing—then it was feared he could use them to work magic against the person to whom they belonged. And so the aura of magic and power already surrounding the living hair was extended in superstition and folklore to hair separated from the head, making it the most highly prized and highly feared fetish object of all.

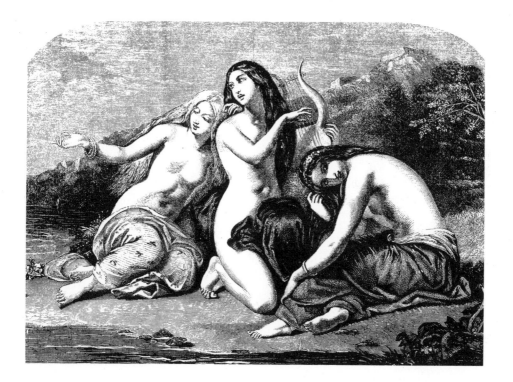

Left: J. Toorop (1858–1928), an artist obsessed with the beauty and sensuality of women's hair, creates strange, erotic patterns with the flowing hair of the women in this painting, The Three Brides. *Above, a 19th-century engraving of the sirens who lured sailors to destruction.*

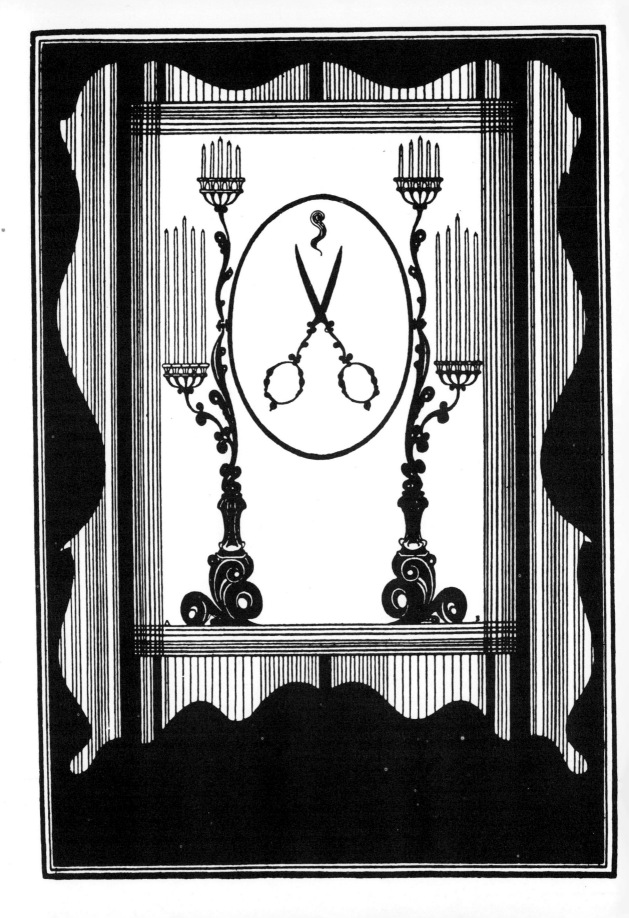

8 *Fear, Fetish, and Favor*

The most simple and direct use of hair as a fetish object has been in the working of magic, for good or evil, by one person upon another. But sometimes even human intervention has been unnecessary; in parts of Europe an old belief still survives that if a bird carries off locks of your hair to build its nest, you will suffer from headaches. To avoid such ill chance, as well as the deliberate machinations of an enemy, it has been the custom in many societies to burn or bury hair combings and clippings or, if they were thought to be needed against the day of resurrection, to hide them carefully from enemies in the meantime.

These practices have been almost universal among primitive tribes throughout the world, though with variations. The Wanyoro of central Africa, for instance, stored all cuttings of hair and nails under a bed, and afterwards scattered them about among tall grass. The Thompson Indians of British Columbia buried or hid loose hair, or sometimes threw it into a river. The Bantu of southern Africa went still further. They not only buried cut hair and nails in a secret spot, but when one of them cleaned the head of another, he carefully preserved any vermin he caught, and politely returned them to their owner. As they had fed upon his blood, the vermin, like the hair, might give an enemy supernatural influence if they fell into his hands.

These superstitions all had their own strange logic. So if the Chilote Indians of southern Chile got possession of the hair of an enemy, they dropped it from a high tree, or tied it to a piece of seaweed and flung it into the surf, confident that the shock of the fall or the thundering of the waves would be transmitted through the hair to the person from whose head it was cut. Similarly, the Marquesan Islanders of the South Pacific

The frontispiece by Aubrey Beardsley (1872-98) to Alexander Pope's The Rape of the Lock *takes as its central motif a pair of scissors and a severed lock of hair—a motif that might be the badge of the true hair fetishist.*

would bury the hair of an enemy, wrapped in an especially intricate way, and the victim would waste away with sickness, unless the hair was discovered and dug up again.

Not only primitive minds were influenced by such ideas. At Rome the *flamen Dialis*, the priest devoted to the service of Jupiter, was subject to many kinds of taboos, and was obliged to bury the cuttings of his hair and nails under a fruit tree. The Greek philosopher Pythagoras, in the sixth century B.C., warned against the danger of standing (even accidentally) upon one's hair clippings, and elsewhere advised spitting upon them as a safeguard. Spitting three times on hair combings before throwing them away was believed at one time to counteract their magic power.

In civilized Europe superstitions about hair clippings survived from generation to generation and from century to century. With as much fervor as the primitive tribes of Africa and elsewhere, the peoples of France, Italy, and England carefully disposed of shorn hair to keep it out of the hands of witches and sorcerers. They also built up a set of superstitions that used hair to cure sickness by a technique of transference. Gout, for instance, could be transferred from a man to a tree by clipping hair from the sufferer's legs, adding nail clippings for good measure, and stuffing them all into a hole bored in an oak tree. The hole had to be stopped up again and smeared with cow's dung. If the patient was free of gout for three months after all this, it was thought the oak was suffering instead, presumably in stoical silence. In Germany toothache was cured in a similar way, and in England certain oak trees in Berkhamsted, Hertfordshire, were celebrated for curing the ague, though in this instance the process was painful, because the hair was pegged to the tree while still attached to the sufferer's head. A sudden wrench was guaranteed to leave the hair, and the malady, attached to the tree. In Bohemia they preferred the willow tree to the oak as a cure for fever. In Oldenburg, in Germany, the technique worked only if the sufferer breathed three times into the hole before plugging it up.

A variation on the tree as recipient is found in an old British superstition, particularly current in the past in Devon and Scotland, that whooping cough could be cured by putting a hair from the patient's head between slices of bread and butter and giving it to a dog. If the dog coughed while eating it, the whooping cough had been successfully transferred. A rather more antisocial habit in Devon was to give a neighbor ague by burying under the threshold of his house a dead man's hair.

Another use of hair was to control the elements, in particular to produce rain. In Western Australia the natives used body hair, plucking it from their armpits and thighs, and blowing it in the direction from which they wanted the rain to come. In the Australian state of Victoria, the wizard sprinkled human hair into the water if a river was running low, or dropped hair into a fire if he wanted to produce rain. For this reason hair could never be burned in the normal way without risk of a deluge. In the Tyrol region of the Alps, witches were supposed to use cuttings or combings of hair in casting spells to make hail storms or thunderstorms, and at one time in the Highlands of Scotland it was said that no woman should comb her hair at night if she had a brother or husband at sea, because if she did his ship would be lost in a gale.

Quite as ambitious as attempting to influence the elements was the use of hair clippings to influence emotions, especially love. One old saying decreed that a girl could draw her neglectful lover to her by tearing out one of his hairs without his knowledge—not, one would think, an easy matter. Far simpler was the method resorted to by a Jewish wife, who would serve her husband with a special pudding whose ingredients included clippings from her hair and nails: this was not expected to do much to whet his appetite for food, but was supposed to do a lot for his appetite for love. Proceeding into the realm of the macabre, a method prescribed in Irish folklore required that a lover obtain a hair from the loved one and run it through the fleshy part of a dead man's leg, to ensure the owner of the hair going mad with love.

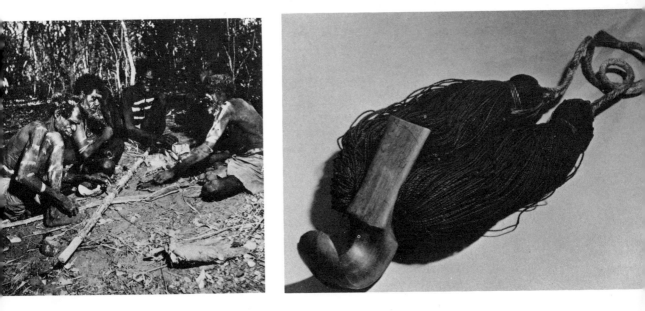

Left, a group of Australian Aborigines making a ritual object (right), constructed of human hair and bone, which they use in their "bone-pointing" ceremony to cause the death of a distant enemy. A belief in the magic power residing in hair is common to many primitive societies.

Such beliefs, with their simple roots in the age-old concept of magic hair, kept a strong hold in earlier times on minds clouded by superstition. To most of us today they seem just unbelievable nonsense. But there is one form of hair fetishism that survives as strongly as ever—the use of hair as a sexual fetish. This derives not from the diminishing influence of superstition, but from the constantly maintained drive of sexuality. To judge from recently published work the practice seems to have increased, but this impression may be due to the fact that modern techniques of analysis uncover sexual aberrations, and modern techniques of communication disseminate them.

The use of hair as a sexual fetish varies from a totally natural admiration for a woman's hair, in which it acts as one stimulant toward sexual excitement and eventual intercourse, to the pathological extreme where individuals find satisfaction in women's hair alone, divorced from their bodies. In such cases the locks of hair are used as means of physical or mental onanism. As long ago as 1785, a German writer, Johann Wilhelm von Archenholz, outlined a classical example:

"I have known an Englishman who was a lovable man of great integrity but who had one most peculiar taste, which, as he assured me, lay deep in his soul. The greatest of pleasures, and the only one which could intoxicate his senses, was to comb the hair of a beautiful woman. He kept a charming mistress for this sole purpose. Love and womanhood did not come into the question at all here. He was only concerned with her hair, which she had to let down at hours which suited him, so that he might rummage in it. So doing gave him bodily pleasure of the highest possible kind."

Emile Laurent, a French penologist and psychologist, confirmed the frequency of this type of hair fetishism with a case he reported in his book *L'Amour Morbide* (1891). He wrote: "One constantly saw at the Bal Bullier in Paris, a tall girl whose face was lean and bony, but whose black hair was of truly remarkable length. She wore it flowing down her shoulders and loins. Men often followed her in the street to touch or kiss the hair. Others would accompany her home and pay her for the mere pleasure of touching and kissing the long black tresses."

A similar but fictitious incident is cited by the English writer John Cleland in the 18th century. In his novel *Fanny Hill*, the heroine, who works in a London brothel, finds satisfying the demands of an elderly client a very easy way of making money: " . . . I let down my hair as loose as nature, and abandon'd it to him to do what he pleased with it; and accordingly he would keep me an hour or more in play with it, drawing the comb through it, winding the curls round his fingers, even kissing it as he smooth'd it; and all this led to no other use of my person, or any other liberties whatever . . . ."

One woman confided to her doctor that, on her wedding night, her husband fumbled with her rather meager tresses and then went off to sleep. The same happened on the following night, but on the third night he produced a wig made up of abundant long hair, and asked her to wear it. Immediately, he was able to make love to her, and she not surprisingly consented to this adornment in bed from then on. Unfortunately the wig was effective for only 15 to 20 days, and so there was a succession of wigs, in all colors, but always long and abundant. At the end of five years the happy couple had two children and 72 wigs.

As one might expect, pubic hair features strongly as a sexual fetish, because of its direct sexual connotations. There is a long history of men collecting pubic hair from women with whom they have had intercourse, and many of them have relived their pleasure by looking at it and handling it. In *Aberrations of Sexual Life,* a book based on the writings of the celebrated German neurologist Dr. Krafft-Ebing (1840-1902), many such cases are outlined, including one where the fetishist found his greatest delight in tearing out hairs from the mons veneris with his teeth. He kept a collection of these hairs and by biting on them again obtained renewed sexual satisfaction. The same man bribed hotel servants to let him look for pubic hairs in beds in which women had slept.

Perhaps the most famous of all cases is that of Christie, the British mass murderer, who in 1953 admitted having killed 11 women. Four sets of female pubic hair, neatly separated and arranged, were found in an old tobacco tin among his other possessions.

Although hair fetishism seems restricted to men, it is not always heterosexual. *Aberrations of Sexual Life* quotes a case of moustache fetishism where a 20-year-old man loved only other men with big moustaches. On one occasion, he met a man corresponding to his ideal and took him home, only to be miserably disillusioned when his visitor took off his artificial whiskers. Only when he was persuaded to put them on again could the affair go forward.

One form of hair fetishism involves the cutting-off of hair, and the act of cutting seems as pleasurable as the possession or handling of it. Cases have been reported in which successful wielding of the scissors has been enough to produce an ejaculation. More often this is obtained by using the hair for masturbation. One 40-year-old bachelor, arrested in Paris after having cut off by force the plait of a young girl, confessed to having done the same thing 10 times before. He admitted having the plaits at home and getting great delight from them. In fact, when his rooms were searched, 65 plaits were found sorted into packets.

Dr. Krafft-Ebing cites another case of a man of high social class, strongly attracted to women's hair from the age of eight, who later suffered agony under the tyranny of plait fetishism. As a young boy he tried to satisfy himself with drawings of plaits, but as an adult found himself in crowded streets either pressing kisses on women's heads or occasionally trying to cut off a plait. Eventually, in his misery he became an alcoholic.

According to Havelock Ellis, this fetish for cutting off hair can be directed to "either flowing hair or braided hair, but is usually one or the other, and not both." Although in Freudian terms the act is seen as a symbolic rape involving some element of sadism, Havelock Ellis, in his *Psychology of Sex,* clearly disagrees with this. He writes: "As a rule the hair-despoiler is a pure fetishist, no element of sadistic pleasure entering into his feelings."

In most people such deviations arouse at worst revulsion and at best pity. But most completely normal instincts are capable of extension in degree and direction, taking them across the borderline of what is acceptable to society. Certainly, throughout history, one of the most normal and universal instincts in man has been to admire human hair. This admiration has often been compounded of both aesthetic and sexual appreciation, and lovelocks and token exchanges of hair have been part and parcel of the ritual of romantic love, far removed from the bewildering and often ugly forces of sexual fetishism.

It is sometimes difficult to know whether hair is being used as a fetish object, a love token, or a trophy. Charles II, for example, is reputed to have owned a wig made up entirely of pubic hair from his many mistresses, and this became the proudest possession of the notorious Wig Club of Edinburgh, a highly erotic 18th-century society. The wig had been taken from another club, Beggar's Benison, whose members began collecting material for a replacement wig to be made from the hair of the mistresses of George IV. Presumably he was not able to rival Charles II in these matters, for it seems never to have got further than a few wisps kept in a snuffbox labeled: "Hair from the Mons Veneris of a Royal Courtesan of George IV." Pubic hair was, of course, exchanged between lovers as a romantic token—for example Caroline Lamb, the wife of the British prime minister Lord Melbourne, sent a gift of her pubic hair to Byron in the course of their brief but passionate affair.

But head hair has been far more often used, and indeed has been the chief love token of all ages. It is interesting to speculate why it should have been singled out in this way. It is not simply that it is more or less imperishable, or that it can be cut and carried with ease. Both fingernails and toenails possess much the same virtues, but lovers have not been notably tempted to use cuttings from these for tender exchanges. Hair, on the other hand, has been cut and exchanged, to be hoarded in caskets, tied up in ribbons, flaunted on hats, secreted next to the heart, borne into battle, and generally used as amulet, favor, keepsake, and *memento mori*.

Quite obviously, there is something about hair that makes it the very stuff of romance. To begin with, it has built-in attraction purely as a physical object. It has color, shape, texture, gloss, and perfume—all calculated to tease the senses and haunt the memory.

But this straightforward physical appeal is further subtly heightened by the lingering aura of magic, myth, and symbolism that still surrounds hair, and quickened by the powerful undercurrent of sexuality it continues to generate. The result is a highly charged emotive object, appealing to the

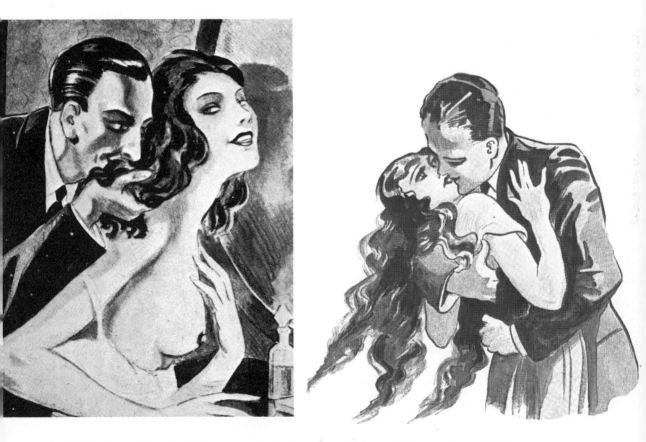

Left, "The Scent of Her Hair," a drawing by W. Plantikow. Right, an illustration from a British magazine, published in the 1930s, catering to hair fetishists. The flowing tresses of the women in these drawings are deliberately exaggerated, just as the breasts may be made more pneumatic in certain types of pin-up—and for precisely the same reason.

sentiment, and rousing the poet, in us all. Just to think about hair in the romantic sense brings words tumbling to the mind: caressing, smooth, silk, satin, gossamer—all crowd in to suggest the feel of hair; flowing, floating, rippling, gleaming, streaming, tossing—all conjure up the sight of hair.

It is small wonder that literature abounds in references, or that hair is second only to eyes as the physical attribute most celebrated and praised by lovers and writers. One of the most famous poems about hair, *The Rape of the Lock* by the 18th-century poet Alexander Pope, manages to fuse together most of the different elements of hair mystique, and is of special interest because it satirizes a real incident.

The actual event involved the 22-year-old Lord Petre, who in an amorous moment rashly snipped off a lock of hair from the head of Miss Arabella Fermor, a famous beauty of the day. Such ill-feeling resulted between the two families that Pope was persuaded to pour poetic oil onto troubled social waters. In fact, his brilliant libation only stirred up more storms, because his parody mocked the seriousness with which the relatively innocent prank was being treated by endowing the stolen lock with the Greco-Roman symbolism of virginity. His Baron raped, if not the heroine Belinda's actual virginity, at least the ritual outward sign and badge of it,

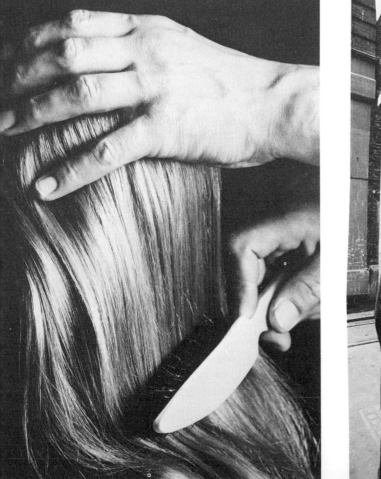

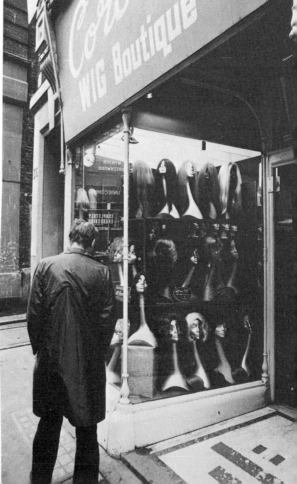

the totemic lock by which her maidenhood was recognized in society.
Clearly it was the ruination not of her coiffure but of her reputation that
made poor Belinda exclaim in anguish:

Oh hadst thou, Cruel! been content to seize
Hairs less in sight, or any hairs but these!

As well as the sexual symbolism, Pope in his poem recognized the sexual
attraction and power of women's hair to enslave men:

Love in these labyrinths his slaves detains,
And mighty hearts are held in slender chains.
With hairy sprindges we the birds betray,
Slight lines of hair surprize the finny prey,
Fair tresses man's imperial race insnare,
And beauty draws us with a single hair.

Shakespeare, in similar vein, made Bassanio in *The Merchant of Venice*
exclaim about Portia's portrait:

. . . Here in her hairs
The painter plays the spider, and hath woven
A golden mesh to entrap the hearts of men,
Faster than gnats in cobwebs.

But it is loose, flowing hair that seems always to have most stimulated
Man's desire and to have been most depicted in his poetry. The Byzantines,
with their direct and joyful acceptance of erotic pleasure, placed great
emphasis on the sensual role of hair. Paul, a sixth-century Byzantine
poet, describes the effect of his mistress's hair on him, especially when it
was unbound:

When loose your tresses lie
And o'er them softly drawn
A neckerchief of lawn
Protects them from men's eyes,
While all in vain my gaze I turn,
My thoughts with longing madly burn.
But when those locks revealed
Send down their stream of gold
And in my hand I hold
Their splendour unconcealed,
No more I feel my heart my own,
A fugitive from reason's throne.

Ovid was clearly aware of the importance of hair in arousing desire, for
in his poem *The Art of Love* he warns women: "Don't neglect your hair,"
and goes on to give lengthy advice on how to dress it to suit each individual

*Hair fetishism is a matter of degree. It is perfectly normal for a man to find erotic enjoyment in
touching, caressing, or brushing a woman's hair (far left). But the man gazing at a display of long
and luxuriant women's wigs in a shop window (left) is perhaps one step farther along the road to
true hair fetishism.*

face. But even more revealing than this are the lines in which he scolds his own mistress for burning her hair with bleaches. He softens his words, however, with praise:

> My dear, your hair was perfect:
> delicate to touch;
> one feared to braid it—it was as fine as silk,
> finer than silks that dark-skinned girls from Asia
> wear at a feast,
> and fragile as the spider's silver thread,
> its colors dazzled, neither black nor gold,
> of that rare light,
> that breaks through shadows of a spring-freshed valley,
> and of the bark-stripped cedars on the hill.
> And never twice the same;
> it fell a hundred ways, in waves, in ripples,
> nor comb's teeth tore it—
> docile it was, and bright, and never angry,
> so girls who dressed your hair never fear it—
> nor hairpin scratched their arms—
> my girl as gentle as her cheerful hair.
> So I have seen her of an early morning,
> languid and naked,
> serene as sunlight on her purple bed,
> her hair in charmed disorder at one shoulder. . . .

Love poems of Elizabethan England also lavished praise on women's hair. Robert Tofte wrote of:

> . . . golden tresses loose (a joy to see!)
> Which gentle wind about thy ears doth blow.

In return for poetic praise and adoration, a lady was expected to bestow some small gift as a sign of favor. Robert Burton, author of the *Anatomy of Melancholy,* refers to this practice: "If he get any remnant of hers, a busk-point, a feather of her fan, a shoo-tye, a lace, a ring, a bracelet of hair, he wears it for a favour on his arm, in his hat, finger, or next his heart."

Even earlier than the 17th century there are records of locks of hair being given as love tokens. They were carried into battle at Agincourt (1415), and throughout the Middle Ages they were exchanged as a pledge of faithfulness to a contract, friendship, or love.

Not unnaturally, if a love affair went wrong the love token often suffered. From the 17th century the story has come down of the lock of hair given by Venetia Stanley to Sir Kenelm Digby, her childhood lover.

This tall and handsome nobleman was a favorite of Charles I and was sent by him to escort the king's bride, Henrietta Maria, from Paris. When he fled abroad again to escape a forced marriage to an heiress, he took with him the lovelock that Venetia had bestowed upon him, only to fling it into the fire when he heard rumors that she was to marry someone else. Venetia, who seems to have led an interesting life, had certainly been abducted by one nobleman and rescued by another, but her engagement to her rescuer, Sir Edward Sackville, came to nothing. Later, back in London, Sir Kenelm met Venetia again, and their old passion was rekindled. He attempted to seduce her, and ended by marrying her. History does not say whether she was generous enough after the reconciliation to spare him another lock of hair.

Even great soldiers could become romantic about hair. The first Duchess of Marlborough, who had a fierce temper, one day—during a quarrel with her husband, the victor of Blenheim in 1704—cut off the beautiful long hair she knew he loved. Returning to the room after a typically melodramatic exit, she found the locks of hair gone, and only years later, when she was sorting through her husband's effects after his death, did she come across them again. The poor duchess related this tale many times afterwards, and wept copiously at every telling.

The lock of hair that the English essayist William Hazlitt received from Sarah, a lodging-house girl he passionately loved, suffered exceptionally harsh treatment. In his book *Liber Amoris,* published in 1822, Hazlitt describes his frenzy when Sarah went off with a young man more appropriate to her station. "I tore the locket which contained her hair (and which I used to wear continually in my bosom as the precious token of her dear regard) from my neck and trampled it in pieces." Later, after screaming and raising the whole household, he "gathered up the fragments of the locket of her hair which were strewed about the floor, kissed them, folded them up in a sheet of paper and sent them to her with these lines written in pencil on the outside: 'Pieces of a broken heart, to be kept in remembrance of the unhappy. Farewell!' "

Far more moving than the histrionics of Mr. Hazlitt was the more practical tone of James Power, an ex-Trappist monk, who loved and lost Julia Woodforde in the 19th century. He wrote to her: "I purchased yesterday a diamond mourning ring: I will place a braid of your hair and mine in it. On the inside I will inscribe: 'James T. Power, died—', leaving a vacancy for the date; if this should be my fate shortly, you will receive an account of the time and get it filled up and I have no doubt you will regard the ring with affection and wear it on my account. You will consider this a romantic proceeding, anticipat'ng what may not happen. Very true. Please send me a small lock of your hair to place in it as soon as possible." But it did happen. The young man died at sea on his way home to England from Sierra Leone in 1819. And the dashing Julia, who had helped the young monk to escape from his monastery, but whose father had not approved the match, died in 1873 a staid spinster, with just a secret bundle of old love letters, and a ring containing her true love's hair.

Sometimes, among acknowledged gallants, lovelocks must have been trophies as much as tokens. Hundreds of locks of women's hair were found among George II of England's possessions at his death. One of them had been sent to him from the deathbed of Perdita Robinson, the actress: and George was described as receiving it "with a strong demonstration of sensibility."

The poet Byron spent only three days in Seville, Spain, staying at the house of two unmarried ladies, but he apparently made such an impression on the elder that at parting she cut off a lock of his hair, and in return presented one of her own—measuring three feet in length. This now resides in the Murray collection of Byron relics at 50, Albemarle Street, London. Byron always insisted that although the lady offered him a share of her apartment, his virtue made him decline. This seems decidedly unlikely, but it may have been discretion, for she was known to be on the point of marrying a fierce officer in the Spanish army.

Another story about Byron involving a hair token, which seems equally in character, is told by the English writer Lord David Cecil in *The Young Melbourne* (1939). It seems that after Caroline Lamb's affair with Byron was brought by the latter to an abrupt end, she bombarded him with alternate threats and pleadings. One of her requests was for a bracelet of his hair. He obliged her, but because he was thoroughly bored and irritated with her, he sent her a bracelet made up from the pubic hair of Lady Oxford (a friend of Byron and Caroline Lamb), who had the same colored hair. He thought this deception a great joke.

It is not just in advanced cultures that hair has been used as a love token. Among the Vedda of Ceylon it was a custom for the bridegroom to present his bride with a lock of hair as part of the wedding ceremony, though if he could not spare it from his own head, he was permitted to take it from his sister's. In Australia, too, locks of hair were exchanged by the aborigines as tokens of affection, and worn around the neck. It was considered unlucky to give away or lose such a keepsake, and among the aborigines of Victoria, if a young girl gave her lover a lock of her hair, it was a mark of the greatest confidence.

An Australian aborigine still leading a Stone Age life could hardly be further from an English girl of the 19th century, yet the prim Victorian miss who pledged her love with a lock of her hair was behaving in exactly the same way. She would no doubt have been shocked to know it, but she was responding to the same primitive instinct as she sighed and shed a soft tear over her true love's hair, sending in return a curl to be worn in a locket or ring, or to be intricately woven into a watch chain. The Victorian age saw the peak of hair sentiment and art. It was as though an age conditioned to be ashamed of sex compensated by indulging in sentiment. While sex was brushed under the carpet, sentiment was worn on the sleeve. It was a period when even piano legs were considered provocative enough to require a cover of frills for modesty's sake. Ankles were indelicate, knees indecent, thighs unmentionable, and bottoms concealed by bustles. As a result, the shoulders, the neck, and the crowning glory of hair became the respectable focus of sexual interest, the acceptable substitute for all the rest. Hair came into its own as one part of the person that it was perfectly permissible to gaze upon and openly adore. And so sentimental interest centered more than ever before on hair tokens in a wide variety of forms.

Such sentiment has always been open to commercial exploitation and hair sentiment was no exception. Two advertisements of the period are fairly typical. The first in 1847 read:

> Important to Ladies wishing to preserve the Hair of a Relative or Friend. Mr. DEWNEY wishes to state that he is a WORKING ARTIST and that hair entrusted to him does not leave his possession until made and returned in the form desired. An Elegant Hair and Gold Ring 3/6d; fine guard ditto 5/6d.

In 1852, under the heading "Hearts United," the following appeared:

> Hair Rings, lined throughout with good solid gold and
> two gold hearts united upon, with the initials.................. 5/6d.
> The same, with two gold hands united in place of hearts...... 7/6d.

Hair was not only incorporated into rings, bracelets, brooches, purses, lockets, and the like, but gradually developed into an art form in its own right. From the simple embroidery of initials in hair on handkerchiefs and sets of linen, the idea was extended to include whole pictures worked in hair. At the Great Exhibition in London in 1851, likenesses were displayed, worked in hair, of Queen Victoria, Prince Albert, and all the royal children. Beneath them were emblems of Church and State, the army and navy, the arts and sciences, commerce and industry, all executed in hair in minute and perfect detail. Family memorials were worked in the same way, with perhaps a scroll of feathers, each separate feather being worked in the hair of one member of the family.

Hair flowers were made, too, sometimes fashioned into a family wreath, with each member having a flower or part of a flower made from his or her hair. Often, a husband's and wife's hair were combined in one flower, with the longer hair of the wife making the petals, and the husband's hair from head or beard forming the center. These wreaths were framed and hung on the wall, or sometimes the hair flowers were formed into a tree and kept under a dome-shaped glass. The fashion was popular on both sides of the Atlantic, as was that for watch chains made from hair.

Since those days, two world wars have seen separated lovers still seeking comfort and reassurance in locks of each other's hair. In the mud of Flanders many a man felt for a moment less lonely as he held in his hand a few strands of bright hair. And a quarter of a century later, among the young pilots flying to challenge the enemy in the skies over England, there were some who carried a lock of a girl's hair with them, as earlier fighters had done riding their horses to Agincourt.

Now, of course, at least for the time, it seems as if sentiment is out and sex is in. No one could wish back again the hypocrisy and double standards of Victorian times, but in banishing them it would be a pity if we banished too the gentler arts of love. Do young men write to ask their girls for locks of hair today as poor Mr. Power did a century and a half ago? For that matter do they write at all in these days of instant communication and instant love?

But one thing at least is certain, looking at the young, at the interest they show in each other's hair styles, at the shining healthy hair of the girls, and at the lion's-mane display of the young men, it is obvious that hair continues to exert its age-old attraction and to fulfill its basic sexual role.

Will it always be so? It has taken three billion years of evolution to produce man and to modify him to his present form, with more brain and less hair. Where will he go from here, assuming that he is not destroyed by the potent mixture of old aggression and new technology? More particularly, where will his hair go from here?

Apart from the instant accident of a mutation, evolutionary changes are so slow as to be imperceptible in the short term. Certainly over the whole period of recorded history we can detect no change—much less a dramatic one—in the distribution or extent of human body hair, despite its decreasing importance as a sexual cynosure with the coming of clothing.

As far as head hair is concerned there is some evidence that the incidence of baldness has increased, at least among urban men subjected to the stress

Opposite, a folk cure for whooping cough—a sandwich made from the sufferer's hair and fed to a dog—and a fetishist's treasure—a collection of women's pubic hairs. Overleaf: left, a wooden shield of the Kenyah tribe of Borneo decorated with locks of hair from slain enemies; right, a mask worn by Balinese dancers, embellished with human hair, and representing a malign female spirit. On page 231; the hair remains grotesquely rich and lustrous on a shrunken human head.

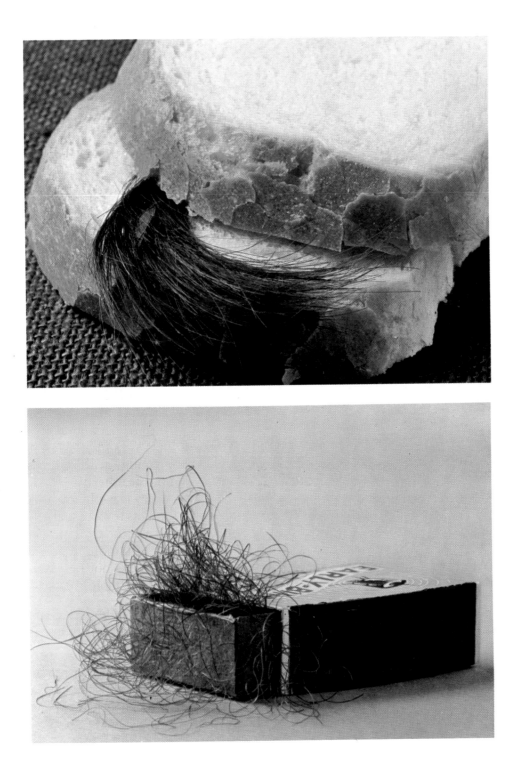

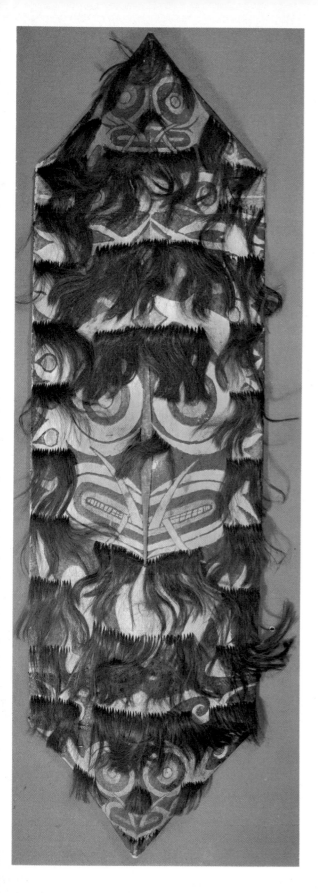

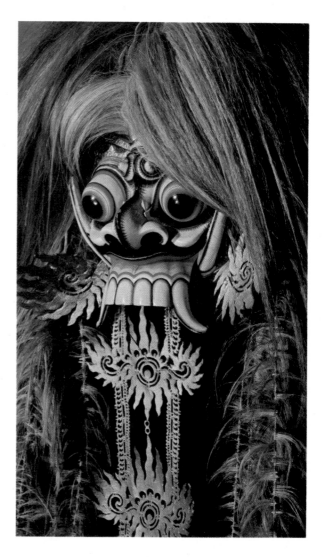

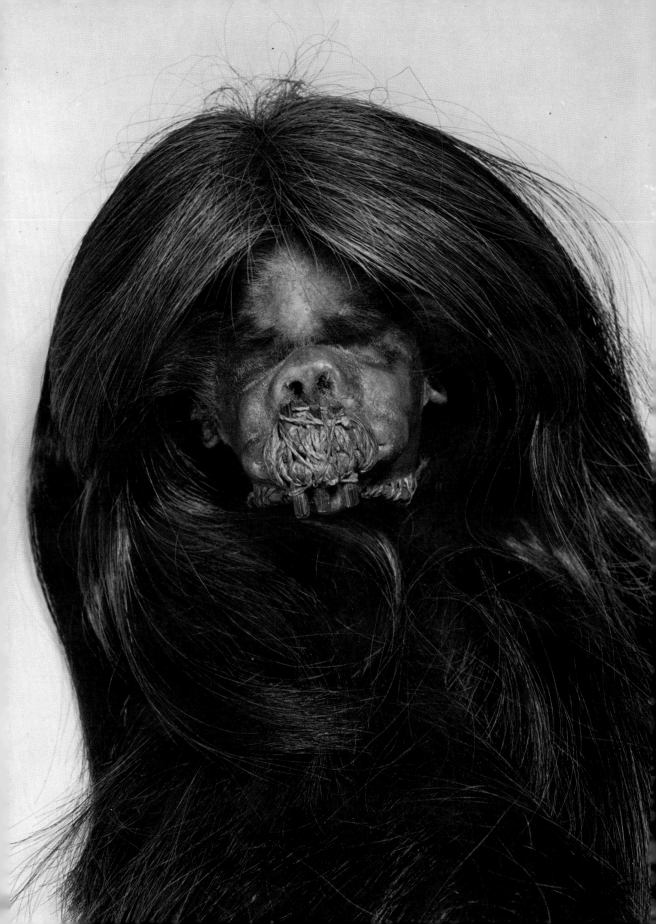

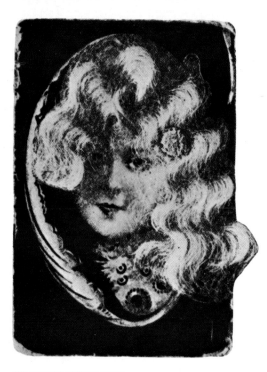

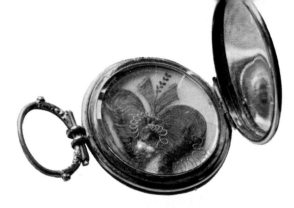

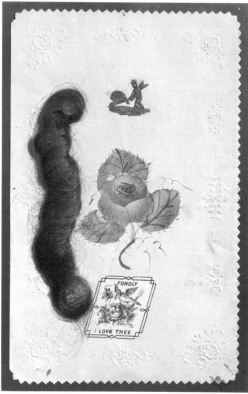

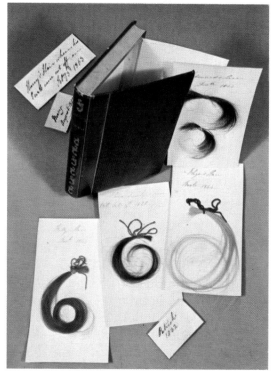

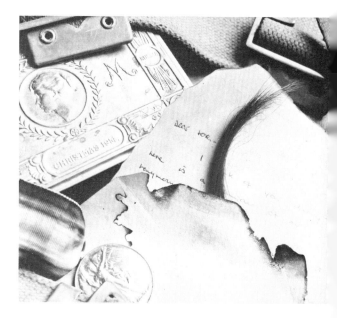

factors of modern high-density living. And there are some indications that women are becoming increasingly prone to baldness, presumably because as they take on a more masculine role they fall victim to the tensions and traumas that go with it. These tendencies are admittedly slight, but they become more significant when seen against their modern background of better hygiene, better general health, and better hair care—which should produce more luxuriant rather than sparser locks.

This tendency toward increasing baldness, if it is confirmed over the centuries to come, we should expect to be gradually assimilated into a transmitted genetic factor. We should expect our descendants to become increasingly prone to baldness. But new and startling developments in the biological sciences now have to be taken into account. With our advancing knowledge in the field of cellular and genetic engineering, natural evolution may never again be allowed to determine unaided our future shades, shapes, peculiarities, and potentialities. It will be within man's scope, if he wishes, to participate increasingly in drawing up the blueprints for his own species.

In the face of our present inability to control our existing technology for the common good, such possibilities are more frightening than reassuring. But they could mean eventually that man will be able to eradicate adverse factors from his own chromosomes. If, for example, he continues to find hair attractive and to desire to keep it in all its glory throughout his life, then the possibility is there. He will ultimately possess the skill to whittle the baldness gene out of the chromosome. Or, if a particular physical type of beauty became the desired ideal, it would be possible to produce it. The factors for blue eyes and fair hair, for example, could be introduced to the chromosome and, over a long period, the gene pool could be influenced toward more and more blue-eyed fair-haired offspring, with ultimate conformity to the pattern. It may, eventually, even be possible to go beyond this and breed individuals to order, to produce a blonde bombshell or a black-haired beauty on demand.

But such science-fact theory is still hundreds of years ahead of science-fact practice, and for the moment we must be content to struggle along in all our glorious and inglorious diversity, treasuring our hair, postponing its premature loss by good hygiene, and camouflaging its ultimate fall with the latest thing in hair weaving, wigs, pieces, or transplants.

The world about us will change, our skills and technology continue to improve, but human nature changes little, and there seems no doubt that, as far into the future as we can see, man will go on responding to the fascination of hair and using its power, sexually and socially, as he has always done.

A collection of sentimental relics and love tokens: top left, a Victorian Valentine with real locks forming the girl's hair and, bottom left, a 19th-century home-made American Valentine decorated with a tress of the sender's hair; top right, a Victorian locket containing a lock of a loved-one's hair; center right, a dummy volume—also Victorian—containing carefully mounted locks of hair from each member of a family; and, bottom right, some mementos of World War I, with a soldier's letter enclosing a lock of hair.

Index

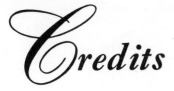

Credits

Key to picture positions: (T) top
(C) center (B) bottom; and
combinations, e.g. (TL) top left
(BR) bottom right.